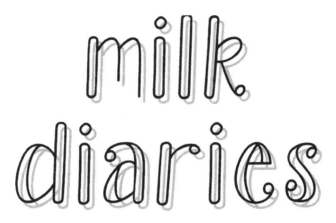

milk diaries

*a compilation of practical, encouraging
advice from the "real" breastfeeding experts*

maggie singleton

ISBN 978-0615671024

Printed in the United States of America.

Cover photograph: © 2009, The Boppy Company, LLC. All rights reserved. Used with permission.

CK Simplicity font used courtesy of Creating Keepsakes Scrapbooking Magazine – www.creatingkeepsakes.com.

Graphics on dedication page and at the beginning of each chapter courtesy of Tagxedo.com.

Definitions at the beginning of each chapter courtesy of Merriam-Webster online dictionary – m-w.com.

This book is intended as a reference volume only. The information is designed to help you make informed decisions about your health and the health of your baby. It is not intended as a substitute for any treatment that may have been prescribed by your physician. If you suspect that you or your baby has a medical issue, please seek competent medical help.

The names of some contributors have been changed as requested.

Internet addresses provided were accurate at the time of publication.

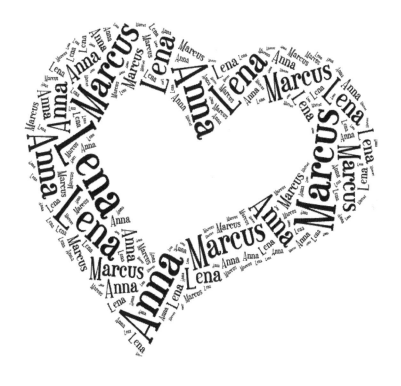

This book is dedicated to my three children.

You have brought me great joy, unforgettable memories,

and a whole lot of lessons learned.

Foreword

Now I need to be honest with you right from the beginning. I'm not a breastfeeding expert. I'm not even a lactation consultant. I'm just a typical mom who decided to give breastfeeding a whirl. And despite all of the classes I took and self-help books I pored over, that's not where I discovered the secret to breastfeeding success. Success isn't lurking in the perfect latch or determined by how much milk you can make. It's not even measured by how long you decide to breastfeed. Instead, "successful" breastfeeding lies in your heart, in your will, and with a great deal of encouragement from your friends and family. (Of course, having your body cooperate is a big plus!)

I thought I was simply making the more healthful, cost-effective choice when I decided to breastfeed. What I didn't realize is how that single decision would affect every facet of my life. All of a sudden you are not only caring for a new baby, you are basing your entire life (what you eat, what you drink, when you sleep, what you do—everything) around this hungry little bundle.

So why do I bring up these disadvantages in the midst of trying to encourage you to breastfeed? I bring them up so you understand that it IS difficult. It IS a lifestyle. It IS a commitment. But once you transcend those truths, you can embrace the challenges and face them head on.

And I'll let you in on my little secret, my source of power, when facing these challenges: my girlfriends. Just as they shared their trials and tribulations of pregnancy and delivery, they were there through breastfeeding too. And they all had a different perspective. I hope you appreciate the following stories as much as I have enjoyed the support I received from the women behind them.

Whether you plan to nurse for one week or two years, you will hit bumps (and lumps, and hiccups, and perhaps some unfortunate clogs) along the way. That's when you'll need characteristics like determination, humor, wisdom, and confidence to ensure breastfeeding success. For that reason, I have broken this book down into four sections, with stories that fit each of those characteristics. You can read the book from start to finish; or if you need encouragement dealing with a particular problem, you can jump to that section to find the type of encouragement you need. There is also a glossary and index in the back to guide you through even more specific needs.

I hope the sound advice from seasoned veterans helps you make decisions that are right for you and your family; and that these stories are a constant encouragement to you throughout your breastfeeding journey.

Table of Contents

Acknowledgements

"A friend is someone who knows the song in your heart and sings it back to you when you have forgotten the words." (author unknown)

I forgot the song in my heart while I was writing and compiling this book more often than I'd care to admit. I cannot thank my friends enough for helping me remember not only my words, but also their own.

Of course, I have had a wonderful friend who has been right there from the moment I said, *some day I'm gonna write a book.* Andy, you have supported me in so many ways...through endlessly holding our firstborn in the middle of the night when we began this thing called parenthood—to watching our now three kids on many occasions so I could steal away to write— to reviewing the book not once, not twice, but three times to help me get everything "just so." Thank you for your love, encouragement, and sense of time management!

Obviously I owe a HUGE thank you to all the moms who contributed a story. Your words took time away from your hectic schedules, and yet you still willingly shared your voices, your stories, your hearts in an effort to help other moms. A special thank you to my "cabin friends." I couldn't make it without your friendship, listening ears, and encouraging words.

Deidre, if you hadn't shared your milk diary with me—how Paul would work the pump *for* you when you were unable to do it yourself (what a trooper)—this book idea may never have been born. I have thoroughly enjoyed getting to know you better through Mothers of Preschoolers (MOPS), and I thank the entire MOPS organization for empowering me to see my goal through to the end.

(I'm sneaking in this section now that my editing team has combed over the book.) Words cannot describe my gratefulness to Kelly Suellentrop, Mindy Windholz, Karyl Iffrig, and Melissa Dereberry for taking the Humpty Dumpty ~~ruff~~ rough draft I gave you and putting it back together again. Thank you!

I feel like this acceptance speech is going to get cut off any minute, so before it does, I also want to thank K.C. White for putting together a lovely website as well as providing terrific advice; Legal Joe for giving me some much-needed legal consult; Tom Petersen for helping me create a smashing logo; Kate Devlin, Cindi Rapp, and Meg Heitlinger from the Boppy Company LLC for allowing me to use a graphic on the front cover; and Nikki Bess for making my mug shot look like a glamour shot. You all are the best!

Lastly, I have to thank my mom for being the first and best nursing "expert" I ever knew!

My Story

As our third and youngest got older, it was time to rid ourselves of all things baby. However, I just couldn't part with my Boppy® pillow. It signified a year in the life with each of my kiddos...three seasons that sometimes seemed like they would last forever and at other times passed in a blink of an eye.

But I am on the other side of perspective and for some of you just beginning this journey, it's difficult to see the light at the end of the tunnel. That's why I decided to write this book. I needed all the encouragement and wisdom and success stories I could get when first starting out—especially with my Lena.

Before our first daughter was born, my husband and I took several classes to prepare for the transition to parenthood. We went through Lamaze, Breastfeeding 101, CPR, you name it. I also attended several La Leche League (LLL) meetings where I met a handful of moms who were already doing what I planned to do. It just seemed to be the most practical way to feed my baby since I'd be home with her anyway, not to mention the myriad of potential health benefits for the both of us.

I came home from those LLL meetings full of knowledge and wisdom from seasoned vets; but I also found myself overwhelmed because the task of raising a child became so real to me. I was going to have to wake up—several times—in the middle of the night to tend to my baby. I may not finish anything off my "to do" list. I may not even have time to take a shower...for days! As I listened to their stories, I couldn't help but think I could surely do it better than *they* did. I wouldn't need to sleep while baby slept and I could easily keep up my part time editing job because *I* was different! Seriously, how hard could tending to a baby be? How hard could nursing be?

Boy did I eat some humble pie when I got my Lena. My "how hard could this be?" quickly turned into, "how am I ever going to do this?!"

Fortunately, I had a handful of girlfriends and a supportive husband to help.

Soon after Lena was born, I developed an unbelievably itchy rash. The oatmeal baths and Gold Bond weren't cutting it, but I didn't want to take antihistamines or antibiotics for fear they would affect my milk supply. Perhaps I should have taken that risk because it finally got so bad that I was prescribed prednisone. Prednisone has two main side effects: it makes you alert and it makes you ravenously hungry—and it is *definitely* expressed in breast milk! So not only was *I* alert and hungry, Lena was alert and hungry, too. Day and night. Ironically, I had wanted an alert baby, so I guess this was just God's way of answering my prayer? [Note to self: be careful what you wish for...you just might get it!]

We were also faced with another breastfeeding challenge. Lena was often inconsolable (especially at night) unless I was nursing her or we had a loud vacuum cleaner humming right beside her for white noise. It was difficult to determine if it was something I was eating or if it was colic. I went through a great deal of food trials on the off chance that it was something I was passing on to her. A good friend let me borrow her copy of The Fussy Baby Book: Parenting the Fussy Baby and High-Need Child by William and Martha Sears that contained an extensive elimination diet to follow. It also contained a chart that helped us differentiate between a colicky baby and a high-need child.

A bland diet only tasted good for so long, and I never did find the culprit. It was official: Lena had colic. I felt so helpless and inadequate that I couldn't keep my own baby from crying. It was also very isolating. I didn't want to take her out for any length of time for fear that she would wake up and begin squalling. Fortunately I had a wonderful neighbor who had a baby boy just a month older than Lena. We would take stroller walks in the warm outdoors laced with white noise and share our war stories of nursing, dirty diapers, and sleep deprivation. I'm honestly not sure I would have made it without her.

The impressive milk supply I had after Lena first came home from the hospital (can you say Double D!?) soon waned under the pressure of a colicky baby with a mom on prednisone. I was exhausted from lack of sleep and dehydration. I was not taking good care of myself, and I had not fully realized just how much that affected *both* of us. I was anxious; she was constantly awake and hungry. We were a mess!

At her one month checkup, Lena's pediatrician recommended that I supplement with some formula, suggesting that I try to feed her a bottle *first* and then offer her my breast. I must admit that after the brief blow to my ego I was relieved to know that she would accept the formula, she was being fed, and I could get a little break! That is until I realized my milk supply wasn't getting any better; it was actually getting worse. (I suspect pediatrician sabotage. This was the same lady who told me there was no such thing as colic.)

I was bound and determined not to quit despite this setback. In an effort to reestablish a good supply, I contacted my hospital's lactation consultant. She explained that I would need to offer my breast *first* and then supplement, not the other way around. I would also need to pump between meals to stimulate more milk production. Makes perfect sense, right? Believe me, the concept makes so much more sense now that I'm not sleep deprived.

A wonderful friend of mine let me use her double breast pump throughout this ordeal and it made all the difference. With a great deal of gusto, pumping, and fenugreek, my supply was re-established! I also started using a spreadsheet my husband created to chart the frequency and duration of Lena's eating, sleeping, and crying. Eventually patterns emerged and the crying began to decrease while the sleeping began to increase. It was such a sanity saver that I have provided a copy of it on my website, http://www.perspectiveswe.com, as well as on the Milk Diaries Facebook fan page. We used a copy during our hospital stay with the other two, and the nurses loved it!

My rash finally healed, I eventually got off Prednisone, and Lena's colic all but disappeared within four months. And although the time it took to nurse her remained lengthy (most feedings lasting 25 minutes per side), the time between feedings got longer and longer. Lena's sleeping eventually improved, and by the time she was eating solids I was beginning to feel human again. We got out quite often, and I would nurse her just about anywhere. The light at the end of the tunnel was beginning to shine through, and I went on to nurse Lena exclusively until her first birthday.

Things were going so well that we decided to have another! Anna was a whole new ball of wax. In stark contrast to her 6 lb., 13 oz. older sister, Anna entered our world weighing 9 lb., 4 oz. This time around, I prayed for a sleeper; and again, God delivered. She preferred sleeping over eating, and more often than not I would have to wake her up to nurse! Easier said than done. I remember envying other friends who had reported this "problem," and now it was my turn. I would strip her down to a diaper, rub her head in a circular motion, tickle her, you name it. In the end, the best trick I found was to give it time. As she got a few days and weeks older, she would stay awake for longer stints.

Like her sister, Anna took to nursing rather well; unlike her sister, she had a super-strong suck! The unexpected "perk" was that she was finished eating in about 10 minutes flat. I couldn't get her to eat any more. And having a toddler to contend with, I wasn't going to complain. Her eating so quickly did lead to some tummy issues, but that cleared up with some over-the-counter heartburn medicine prescribed by her (new and improved) pediatrician.

And did I happen to mention that Lena took a bottle? Well, Anna only cared for the genuine article. Thankfully she didn't eat for as long because I was the only one who could feed her.

If that was the caveat to having a good sleeper, I would take the good with the bad. But when she was a little older and didn't even take a sippy cup of liquid gold, I began to get nervous about weaning. I had to gradually add more and more breast milk to a sippy cup of juice/water for our little connoisseur. It eventually worked like a charm, and she continued to nurse or take a sippy cup of breast milk until she was a year old.

That brings me to the final chapter of my milk diary. I feel as if my story is like Goldilocks, and Marcus was *just* right. I had heard rumors of boys not figuring out the latch thing as easily. I had heard rumors of them being voracious, aggressive eaters (been there, done that). I wondered how I would possibly have time to nurse him with activities and school schedules to contend with. Thankfully, my worries were just that. My only qualm was how quickly he learned the "I-am-crying-and-need-mommy-to-nurse-me-back-to-sleep" trick. It took a toll on me after a while! (More on that in the Some Habits Die Hard section on page 40.)

My three children brought about three different sets of challenges, and the following pages are packed with lessons I learned along the way. Some of these lessons I gleaned from friends that had already been through a similar situation. Other tidbits are things I wish someone had told me that I ended up learning the hard way. Lucky for you, you'll be ahead of the game!

Lessons Learned

The following little kernels of wisdom are not scientifically tested but they are definitely mother approved—confirmed through a battery of trials I ran on my three favorite test subjects.

Frequent Flier Miles

Think back to the last time you traveled by plane. As part of the litany of precautions before each flight, an airline attendant reminds passengers that, "in the event of a sudden loss of cabin pressure, masks will descend from the ceiling. Grab the mask and pull it over your face. <u>If you have small children traveling with you, secure **your** mask **before** assisting with theirs.</u>" This precaution may seem to fly in the face of mother's intuition, but safety experts realized long ago that you can't take care of your child if you are not taken care of first. This is especially true for nursing moms. You cannot adequately care for your baby if you aren't taking care of yourself. I learned that the hard way!

So put on your air mask first by—

- *Drinking plenty of clear fluids.* Did you know that a dairy cow has to drink 4 gallons of water to produce 1 gallon of milk? Holy cow! That's a lot of water. By no means am I calling you a cow, but I am reminding you to drink...a lot! If your pee is anything but clear, down a glass of water. Have a water bottle or cup handy at various spots around your home as a reminder.

- *Eating right.* Now this can get a little tricky if your baby shows signs of food sensitivity; and I'm all about a little indulgence for breastfeeding moms. But if you're already feeling worn out, don't add insult to injury by *consistently* making poor food choices just because you have an extra 500 or so calories to fulfill.

- *Getting adequate sleep.* Not only is it good for a new mom's body, mind, and spirit; it's also necessary because that's when your body makes more milk! Prolactin, the hormone responsible for milk production, is at its highest levels from 2am-6am. Little cat naps along the way can't hurt either. I know I rolled my eyes when moms reminded me to sleep while baby slept, but it really did make a big difference when I took them up on the advice. You will be able to write thank you cards, clean bottles, work, or finish some laundry more effectively after a good rest.

- *Letting others help whenever and however possible.* I might as well burst your bubble now and let you know about Supermom. It's simply the figment of every mom's imagination. Instead of trying to be Supermom, recognize that you need help and accept it willingly from friends and family. It will make them happy to help, and once you learn to yield that control, you'll be so much better for it. It takes a village (see Gwen's story on page 187).

- *Discovering stress management techniques that work for you.* There is not a doubt in my mind that stress is one of the biggest factors affecting letdown and milk production. This is only compounded by the fact that you have less time and energy to devote to yourself when you're a new mom, and it may be some time before you can resume a normal exercise regimen. So what's a mom to do? You may have to settle for less vigorous activity for a while, but devoting time to yourself doing something completely separate from being a mom can reap big rewards. Some suggestions may include muscle relaxation, singing, meditation, yoga/pilates (although, obviously nothing too exhausting), massage, taking a nice long bath, calling a friend, deep breathing exercises (they aren't just for labor and delivery anymore), journaling or reading (something non-baby related), or helping others.

Sometimes it's the little things that can add up to make you feel the most human again.

Nursing is a Lifestyle

Having had twins just six months before Lena's arrival, my sister knew how demanding infants could be. She wanted to give me the most thoughtful gift she could to help me through those first few weeks: a night off. We enthusiastically hashed out the details of this well-intentioned plan—until it hit me that we had forgotten a rather important detail: I was Lena's sole food source. It was in that moment that I began to realize how nursing was going to be more than a mode of feeding. It was going to be an entire lifestyle shift. It was only in retrospect that I fully realized the amount of sleep I got, my stress level, and what I ate and drank affected my babies and my milk supply. Perhaps it's the all-encompassing nature of breastfeeding that leads some moms to quit earlier than they expected. That's why it's so important to have a goal in mind for how long you intend to nurse (see more on that in the Weaning section starting on page 43).

9 Out of 10 Experts Do Not Agree

Perhaps the second-most burning question on the hearts and minds of nursing moms (right after "is baby getting enough to eat?") is "when is this baby going to start sleeping through the night?" And the answer to that question can be quite dubious. The link between nursing and sleeping cannot be overstated. And a new mom will do just about *anything* to get her baby to sleep—which can lead to some habits that may be hard to break later (more on that in the Some Habits Die Hard section on page 40).

When Lena was a baby, I continued to attend LLL meetings as a way to glean valuable information about nursing as well as a way to get out of the house! I often left those meetings feeling like less of a mom, though, because I hadn't fully embraced the breastfeeding subculture. My daughter loved her binky; I could not figure out how to use a sling to save my life; she wore disposable diapers; and after a brief stint of co-sleeping, we realized it just wasn't working for our family. For *me*, attachment parenting was like trying to fit a square peg in a round hole.

I don't share this experience as a means to criticize other moms. Quite the contrary. I share it to emphasize that there is more than one mothering/nursing lifestyle to choose from, and it's up to you and your family to forge that path. **Neither**

choice is more right or wrong than the other, but it is awfully isolating to think you are somehow not "mom enough" because you don't follow the advice of a popular book or you do things differently than your family or friends.

Consider this decision as a microcosm of your parenting style. Determining what type of nursing mother (and family) you will be sets the stage for future decisions. And the two schools of thought on parenting breastfed babies (attachment parenting and parent-directed feeding...not to mention all the styles that fall somewhere in between) couldn't be more conflicting. Both styles have data to back up their effectiveness—they just go about it in completely different ways.

Attachment parenting is a term coined by Dr. William and Martha Sears and shared in The Baby Book as well as in several other books penned by the dynamic duo. Attachment parenting strives to develop an infant's need for trust, empathy, and affection by creating a secure, peaceful, and enduring relationship. This style requires a consistent, loving, and responsive caregiver—especially during the first few years of life. More often than not this style of parenting involves co-sleeping, on-demand breastfeeding, and little separation from baby. If this lifestyle appeals to you and your family, LLL; The Womanly Art of Breastfeeding; books by Dr. William and Martha Sears (and their sons in some cases); and Elizabeth Pantley's No-Cry Sleep Solution Book can guide you through breastfeeding and sleep.

Parent-directed feeding strives to get baby accustomed to the family's routine—instead of the other way around. The parent-directed method is made up of three basic activities that are repeated in a rhythmical cycle throughout the day: feeding time, wake time, and nap time (note the order). These cycles are both routine and predictable to help baby feel safe and secure.

If you prefer a more structured approach yet still want to exclusively breastfeed, sleeping advice can be a bit more complicated but NOT impossible! First off, I want to make it clear that on-demand feeding is crucial the first month or so of breastfeeding regardless of the long-term lifestyle you choose. I caution nursing moms against any book that recommends stringent ideals about sleeping/eating times.

I prefer Mark Weissbluth's book, <u>Healthy Sleep Habits; Happy Child</u>. It has a section specifically dedicated to breastfeeding and sleep (and I also found it validating and informative with regard to colic). Richard Ferber's book, <u>Solve Your Child's Sleep Problems</u>, is another good read. And although I wouldn't pretend to say she's a big breastfeeding proponent, I also suggest the late Tracy Hogg's book, <u>Secrets of the Baby Whisperer</u>. It contains a very descriptive table to help you decipher different cries so you can respond appropriately to your baby's needs. Her book can also help you establish an E.A.S.Y. schedule (Eat, Activity, Sleep, and You) to add a bit of structure to your day—while making sure you take care of yourself as well as baby.

No matter what lifestyle you choose, take expert opinion with a grain of salt. They do not know your baby nor do they know your particular situation. If you discover an appealing concept (in the books I've mentioned or in the myriad of other sleep books on the market), make sure to stick with it for at least 2-3 weeks. I think part of our sleep issues with Lena stemmed from me growing impatient with one idea and, in a moment of desperation, skipping too quickly to the next possible solution. Our poor little lady never knew what to expect! If you are struggling with this, don't miss Wendy's story on page 151. It puts all the worry about listening to experts in perspective!

Teachable Moments

Breastfeeding does hurt. You try running a marathon without having trained and tell me you aren't raw! Everyone involved in the process is new to the experience. Your nipples will be raw; when your milk comes in, your breasts will be engorged and tender; and it may take a while for your baby to get the right latch; etc. Beginnings are tough, and breastfeeding is no exception.

If the pain continues past a week or your intuition tells you things aren't quite right, seek help from an expert. Most hospital lactation consultants will field calls long after your hospital stay is over. Stores that sell lactation supplies are also a tremendous help. Not only do they sell supplies and provide nursing bra fittings, they often have a lactation consultant on staff who can correct latching techniques, help you through an increase or decrease in milk production, and/or suggest improvements as necessary. Many even have a support group that you can attend or join. There are also a ton of online support groups. See the Helpful Websites section on page 68, Peggy's story on page 75, Amy's story on page 101, and Catherine's story on page 159 for more on breastfeeding pain and seeking help.

Let's Get this Party Started. I had the opportunity to talk to a lot of moms while compiling this book. I was astounded at the number of moms who truly, madly, deeply wanted to nurse their babies and couldn't because "their milk never came in." To be honest, my initial thought was that they didn't give themselves enough time. I do not mean they didn't TRY. I mean they didn't realize that although it usually takes 3-4 days for milk to *really* come in, that it can sometimes take as long as two weeks (in which case supplementation would obviously be necessary).

Experts cite many reasons this can happen...excessive blood loss during labor and delivery...if the entire placenta doesn't pass...inability to get skin-to-skin contact right away after birth. While these are all valid reasons, I would say another big culprit is stress. And, really, who would argue that a mother who just underwent labor isn't stressed? I would contend that all the pressure of fulfilling this one maternal task only a mother can perform—along with all the other stressors that go along with being a new mom—is enough to throw any mom's body out of whack for a while!

Stress can be compounded when drugs are involved during labor and delivery. Although they have not found the drugs themselves to affect breast milk, they can affect the hormones associated with breastfeeding. Some pain medications (especially those used during and after a C-section) elevate dopamine levels which in turn inhibit prolactin's job of making milk. (Those same drugs—used for epidurals and c-sections alike—may also cause you to have flat nipples. See Holly's story on page 141 and Zoë's story on page 193 for more on flat nipples.) Oxytocin, the hormone responsible for letdown, is also affected by stress.

If your milk isn't coming in "right away," there are obviously some things you can do to coax it out. Trying to nurse early and often as well as pumping between attempts will hopefully yield some results. I would also say that cutting yourself some slack for all that your body has just endured, resting whenever possible, and finding ways to relax can go a long way. You aren't Supermom, and that's ok. It will take a village to raise your baby, and it might just take a village to get nursing off to a good start, too. Take a deep breath, accept that it's a tough situation (but one that's hopefully worth getting through), and do what you can. Sometimes your body will slowly but surely cooperate. However, sometimes the advantages will never outweigh the disadvantages and supplementing or completely switching over to formula is the best option. See Peggy's story on page 75, Kelly K's story on page 91, Kelly S' story on page 117, K.C.'s story on page 199, and the Weaning section on page 43 for more on this topic.

Latching. I had always heard that you needed to get baby's entire mouth around your areola to create an affective latch. Therefore, I must have taken Lena on and off my breast about

20 times per feeding in the hospital. OUCH! I was trying to shove my huge areola into her poor little mouth because that's what you are "supposed to do." It simply didn't fit.

As long as your little one's mouth is around most of your areola (and she hasn't wheedled her way down to just your nipple), you can hear the suck/swallow, your breast feels "empty" when baby is finished, and her lips are puckered up, don't sweat it. However if those things are not happening, call in for reinforcements.

Sometimes the littlest changes to position can reap the biggest rewards, too. Make sure that you and baby are belly to belly while trying to nurse. That way she's not craning her neck to eat and your boob isn't being yanked in the wrong direction! See Holly's story on page 141 and Catherine's story on page 159 for more on latching.

Hang Time. I was so proud of my first few nursing sessions with Lena! She just kept eating...and eating...and eating for well over 40 minutes on each side! *Must be some good stuff*, I thought! After she picked her jaw back up off the floor, the kind nurse who came to check on me assured me that Lena could come up for some air. I was merely trying to nurse on demand and nurse often. My breasts did not thank me later for the gesture. And although experts and nurses alike cannot seem to agree on the length of time you should feed baby, 40 minutes per side for the first few feeds is excessive by anyone's standards.

The other question that goes along with hang time is if you should switch sides during a feeding or not. I'd love to tell you the secret to that burning question, but I'm afraid the answer lies not in a book but with you, your child, and a lot of trial and error. With Lena I switched sides halfway through each time; Anna wasted no time and could hardly get through one breast before she would get indigestion; Marcus fell somewhere in between. Is it possible that there's no right answer? Perhaps you can trust yourself well enough to know when baby seems full; or if your boobs are beginning to explode, you can switch sides to alleviate the pressure. You know a lot more about your baby than the experts do! See Kelly S' story on page 117 and Wendy's story on page 151 for some humorous reminders.

One thing is for sure: no matter what timeframe your baby is on, make sure she is getting the hindmilk—the equivalent to a nice, fattening dessert that comes near the end of a feed and provides the calories necessary for her to grow. If your baby doesn't seem to eat as much during a particular meal and gets hungry sooner than the next feeding, nurse her on the same side again so that she gets enough hindmilk.

Engorged! Several of my veteran nursing moms warned me of engorgement like the graduating 2nd graders warned our incoming class about *Mrs. Hellert.* I wasn't really sure what I was in for, but I knew it wouldn't be fun. My breasts had already grown exponentially throughout pregnancy. But that was nothing compared to a day or two after leaving the hospital when I woke up to boobs literally twice the size they were the day before! Under normal circumstances, this would be a dream come true for a barely-B woman such as myself.

Finally! Redemption! Not. so. much. My breasts were painful to the touch and screaming to be popped like a balloon.

Here were the saving graces that got me through engorgement, because BIG boobs + baby's tiny mouth = mounds of frustration:

- I used a hand pump before even attempting to get Lena to latch on the first week or so. (And if that wasn't close enough, squirting some into a nearby sink worked just as well.) The hand pump relieved some of the pressure and made it much easier for her to latch on. If you use this approach, just remember the law of supply and demand. Your body will continue to make that extra 2-3 ounces of milk long after engorgement is over. This can be a blessing for those with low milk supply and a curse for those with an overabundance!

- A friend of mine recommended placing cabbage leaves on my breasts a few times a day to relieve the swelling. While your hubby is at the store filling all your postpartum needs, have him pick up a head of cabbage and you'll be glad you did. Tea leaves are reported to have similar pain-relieving qualities. Just don't overdo it or you may begin to dry up your supply.

- Engorgement should only last a few days while your body is equalizing to meet the needs of baby. That's why consultants are so passionate that you *try* not to supplement at the beginning. They know your body is busy doing some higher-order math to ensure baby gets just the right amount of nutrition in every meal.

- Lastly, in my case at least, engorgement got much less intense with each child.

Breastfeeding is natural? Although breastfeeding is natural, it doesn't always come naturally. It's messy, it's clumsy, and neither person totally knows what's going on at first. Cut yourself and your baby some slack and realize that, just like anything else worth trying in life, it's gonna take some practice to make progress.

For instance, I remember *trying* to nurse my 5-day-old Anna under a blanket at a formal MOPS event. Thank goodness it happened in a room full of moms because it was loud, clumsy, and probably more revealing than I had anticipated. To top it off, she spat all of it up on me seconds later. *So much for wearing a nice outfit.* I've been there and so has every other mom who has tried—regardless of how "natural" it may appear to a novice.

It may take a few trips to a semi-secluded area to feel comfortable nursing in public, but you'll get there. Consider bringing a breastfeeding friend (BFF) along for good measure. I know having my friend Liz sit with me in the corner of our local Panera Bread—me with a blanket over my shoulder fumbling with a newborn and her running interference— significantly helped me feel more comfortable with the idea. It was so refreshing to escape my four walls!

Growth Spurts! Growth spurts are a 2-5 day span when baby eats incessantly. They'll *usually* occur at the following times in the first year: 7-10 days after birth, 6 weeks, 3 months, 6 months, and 9 months. (Those timeframes may vary for preemies or late-comers.) Baby will want to "cluster-feed" (group several meals together), eat longer meals, and may be fussier than normal.

Give in to your baby's needs during this time and don't give up! If you are exclusively nursing, keep it up without supplementing if at all possible. There's a scientific change occurring wherein baby needs more milk to help her grow. Furthermore, your milk is actually changing and you'll begin to make more for your (now) larger baby. Drink clear fluids even more than usual and get as much rest as possible. Your "treat" at the end of the spurt will be a day or two when baby sleeps incessantly.

When You Gotta Go, You Gotta Go. I must say one morning I was actually thankful for those lovely monster feminine pads you get to wear postpartum. It was a middle of the night feed, and I could tell my little guy was HUNGRY. I rushed in to feed him, and as Murphy's Law would have it, that's precisely when I was hit with the urge to pee like a racehorse. I had tried the take-the-whole-Boppy® pillow-and-baby-with-me-to-the-bathroom approach with limited success in the past. But this time, I *really* had to go.

The rest is history. All I can say is thank goodness for those monster pads. They can hold a lot!

Especially at the beginning, you'll be nursing baby quite often at all hours of the night. If your baby is sleeping in a separate spot than you, make sure you *go* pee before you *go* in to see him. The reason is two-part: it's nearly impossible to relax and have your milk come down when you're busy holding in your pee. Also, if you take the time to go to the bathroom, you won't be rushing in at baby's every peep, which might just allow him time to fall back to sleep on his own.

The Isolation Chamber. No joke...when we first came home from the hospital with Lena, my loving, well-intentioned husband made sure all the blinds were shut and put towels across every opening to our front-facing windows so no one could sneak a peek while I was nursing. Despite his thoughtful attempt at modesty, I was suffering from a BAD case of claustrophobia. Having just left a hectic full-time job (completing my last major project while in labor, thank you very much) to begin motherhood was isolating enough. After about two weeks, the blinds were open and the towels came down for good.

Make sure you're getting out (without baby, if possible). If you're unable to physically leave your home, at least get some fresh air. Once you've already gotten some rest while baby naps, visit some forums or blogs to realize that you are far from the only mama going through similar challenges. Make sure you don't lose your sense of you just because you happen to be caring for a wonderful extension of you day in and day out.

Don't Play the Martyr! Sacrifice is something you rarely hear about in American pop culture. The "I want it all and I want it now" way of life comes in stark comparison to one of the most natural, selfless acts you can do for your child. It's that constant sacrifice that can sometimes lead to feelings of bitterness and resentment—at least it did for me.

At times, I wished I weren't the only one who could feed my baby in the middle of the night. At times I wished I could get away from it all for a day—no strings attached. Perhaps I bought into American pop culture more than I thought! Despite an incredibly supportive husband, resentment would build up as a result of the all-encompassing task of nursing our babies. I was mad that he could continue to work out or go ride his bike for hours at a time. I was mad that he "got to" go to work every day. I was even mad that he could go out and mow the lawn all by himself—without worrying about what time it was or when the next feeding would be or how dehydrated he might get as a result. Oh, how I longed to mow that lawn!

Again, he really is a terrific dad and hubby. It was my resentment, not his. It required a great deal of openness, honesty, and collaboration to ward off those feelings. In (eventually) talking with him about it, we worked through it. He found ways to help I hadn't really considered. And with each baby, he seemed to understand more and more how taxing the mere act of nourishing our babies could be. But it took open communication from both ends (not magical mind reading) to get to that point.

So don't be a martyr! Talk openly and honestly with your friends and family and weigh your options. Although it may not seem like it at the time, there are *always* options. And you realize (usually in retrospect) what a small snippet of time this really is.

Semper Gumby. Something else to remember is flexibility. You and baby will *both* change more dramatically in the next few months than you have in the last 10 years! You may decide that you couldn't possibly go back to work because you want to stay home with your new bundle. On the flipside, you may have had all intentions of staying at home but decide you might just go loco if you did. You may want to bottle feed baby ¾ of the time but junior won't take a bottle. Be ready to change it up as your lifestyle needs shift. Being open to change is paramount and a characteristic that is so very important for motherhood in general. See Sarah's story on page 217 on how to maintain an open attitude about nursing.

Breastfeeding While Sick. Anne Smith wrote a terrific article based upon The American Academy of Pediatrics (AAP's) publication, *The Transfer of Drugs and Other Chemicals into Human Milk,* and Thomas Hale's book, Medications and Mother's Milk. I thought I'd save a few trees and share Breastfeeding Basic's link to the article instead (http://www.breastfeedingbasics.com/articles/when-a-nursing-mother-gets-sick). KellyMom.com also provides an exhaustive list of ailments and proper remedies.

Leaky Pipes. So if you read my story, you know that I usually found myself on the other end of the spectrum and struggled to have *enough* milk at most times during my milking career. That was NOT the case one evening when my husband and I decided to leave the kids with Grandma and Grandpa while we enjoyed a friend's wedding reception. To further set the stage, I will add that for whatever reason, my pump was not cooperating with me and I was unable to make a full bottle before we left.

I was having a wonderful time—finally taking my own advice and getting out for a while. The only problem was my fear of springing a leak at any given moment! Thankfully my mom (who apparently did not suffer from a lack of milk and would always tell me how her milk would come down if she so much as heard another baby crying in a store) taught me a wonderful trick for those times when pads may not be enough or your milk is coming in whether you want it to or not. Ready? Here goes. Simply take the palm of your hand and smash the living daylights out of your boob—thus stopping the letdown process. Just like that, my dress and reputation were preserved! [Please note that this technique should not be used on a normal basis, but it certainly works in a pinch.]

Thrush. Although I didn't develop thrush with Lena or Marcus, Anna and I went through it twice (probably because we didn't completely get rid of it the first time around). Thrush is a harmless, yet pesky yeast infection that nursing babies can develop in their mouths and nursing moms can develop on their breasts. You may notice your baby's tongue is unusually white (like cottage cheese) and it doesn't come off when scraped; she is suddenly rejecting breast milk; she has patchy red diaper rash; and/or she is extra gassy. You may also notice your nipples feeling extra tingly and "burning" a bit during letdown. Thrush could be the culprit, and it will require treatment for <u>both</u> of you to get rid of it. Otherwise, you'll continue to pass "the love" back and forth to one another.

My lactation consultant suggested that it may have been the penicillin I got for Group B strep that instigated the thrush (I didn't get to the hospital in enough time with Lena to get any). Just like any other antibiotic, the penicillin left my body prone to a yeast infection; however, this time it appeared on my nipples. To combat the thrush, our pediatrician prescribed this icky oral Nystatin drug for her and my OB/GYN prescribed a Fluconazole pill in addition to dabbing Nystatin on my nipples. I found the treatment to be an annoying addition to the baby care routine, but thankfully there were no further side effects. See Kelly K's story on page 91 for more on thrush.

Just ensure you complete your doses of medication or else the fungus will come back! Actually, take it a day or two longer to be on the safe side because even when your symptoms fade, an overgrowth of yeast may still exist. Also make sure you are religiously replacing your nursing pads. Lastly, eat yogurt. I ate a ton of yogurt after Marcus was born to try to keep my tract more equalized and was able to ward off the effects of the penicillin before an infection could begin. Yogurt is *always* your friend when taking antibiotics. (Remember that later in life if your kiddos need to take antibiotics, too!)

The Truth about Binkies. I was livid to learn that the nurses were giving Lena a binky in the hospital nursery. The nerve! Didn't they know that pacifiers could be the kiss of death for breastfeeding—not to mention their potential to increase ear infections and cause future dental problems?

Well by week two, when colic had really set, I was willing to accept the potential risks. The binky was one of the few tools left in our toolbox. I could finally hear myself think! Since then, all three of my children both successfully nursed and used binkies; and they definitely knew the difference. I'm not saying you *have* to use a binky; but I am saying that it's not something to swear against.

If it seems like your baby is "eating" all the time, make sure he/she is really eating and not just wanting comfort. (If you want to provide your breast as comfort, that's terrific. If you would rather not, binkies provide an alternative that is rarely confused as a food supplement.) According to Peggy's story on page 75, some pediatricians actually encourage binky use to help babies develop a stronger suck. The AAP also recommends that infants use binkies for naps and night time to reduce the risk of sudden infant death syndrome (SIDS).

You may have to try a few different types and brands before finding one that your baby prefers. My girls liked the Gerber First Essentials® binkie that had a straight nipple shaped more like the real deal. On the other hand, Marcus seemed to like the orthodontic-shaped, silicone type better. Of course, it could have been the cute football design the Nuk® pacifier came in that he liked the most.

The "F" Word. As I shared in my milk diary, I supplemented with Lena because of low milk supply. Anyone with a pulse knows that breastfeeding is best, however, there may be times when you <u>need</u> to supplement. Just try to make this an educated decision between you, your family, and your pediatrician and not a split second decision made in a moment of desperation or frustration. Perhaps you have low milk supply or you have unexpected surgery and you don't have much milk saved. Just realize the law of supply and demand and continue to pump! It helps to know how long you plan to nurse so that this period of time remains supplementation and not weaning. There are plenty of valid reasons for moms to supplement with formula and sometimes when it's necessary to use formula altogether. There are also plenty of reasons moms quit nursing that could probably be resolved with a little help. See the Weaning section starting on page 43 if you're struggling.

Is My Baby Anal Retentive? The weirdest phenomenon happened to Lena. Around four months of age, she literally would not poop for 5-7 days straight! My husband coined it the "poop lottery" because you never knew when you were going to be the "winner" who got to cash in on a very messy diaper. Crazy! I was reassured by several health professionals that it's completely normal for breastfed babies and that it does not signal constipation or cause for concern. If this happens to you, take heart. In her case, she outgrew the stage a couple of months later. (Obviously if it continues or you are concerned, contact your pediatrician to ensure nothing else is wrong.) Very rarely are breastfed babies constipated.

Solids. Just when you think you have this whole breastfeeding thing mastered, you arrive at a new fork in the road: feeding baby solids. This was always an awkward time for me. It almost seemed like contraband to feed my baby REAL food. I wasn't used to portion control or highchairs or re-navigating what baby's mouth and tummy could handle. And when should I feed her? After nursing? Before nursing? At a completely different time? So many questions loomed. Meanwhile, Lena was following my every bite with such intensity that I knew she was ready.

I remember her very first "meal" quite well. It was Halloween night, and we had literally moved to the St. Louis area that morning. We went to visit Grandma and Grandpa, who lived nearby, so they could share in the event. As my pediatrician recommended when first starting on solids, I nursed her beforehand. The reason is two-part: baby is less apt to get frustrated because she's hungry, and it also helps maintain your milk supply (as milk will continue to be baby's primary source of nutrition until around her first birthday).

I recalled my LLL leader saying that fresh bananas were a good food to start baby on, so I mashed one up to smithereens, scooped up the tiniest morsel possible, and held my breath as I offered it to Lena. She miraculously knew just what to do and seemed to love being a big girl!

The story doesn't end there, though. She may have had a successful first meal, but she was up ALL NIGHT telling us about it. Her tummy hurt, and it hurt badly. I later learned (after another call to the pediatrician following repeated middle-of-the-night tummy pains) that certain foods such as bananas, carrots, and applesauce can be very binding, especially to a small baby. IF your child has issues with constipation, remember the "p" fruits: prunes, peaches, pears, and plums do wonders to loosen things up, if you know what I mean. In fact, we started adding prune juice to Lena's rice cereal to strike the right balance. I had learned my lesson and started the other two on cereal first.

Personality + My mother-in-law told me that the way her kids entered the world said a lot about their personalities. For example, my husband was two weeks late—calm, content, and in no rush to begin his new life outside the womb. To this day, he remains a calm, content guy who still takes time to ensure he makes sound decisions.

In retrospect, I can say the same about the deliveries of my three. Remarkably, the ways my kids nursed was like another window into their personalities. Lena was an incessant nurser. She would nurse each side about 25 minutes and want more 1.5 hours later! I realize now that it was all part of her budding personality. She's still our cautious cuddler who thrives on time spent with those she loves the most. On the other hand, her sister Anna was a barracuda who would be finished nursing in ten minutes flat. She remains our more impulsive go-getter. Marcus fell somewhere in between—not too fast, not too slow—although I must say that he was the one who "played" with his food source to learn how it all worked more than the girls ever did. Perhaps he'll be an engineer like his Daddy someday.

I'm not sure I would have been afforded the same opportunity to witness their personalities unfold so early if I had not breastfed them. What a gift!

'Til the Cows Come Home. The kids and I decided to go to Purina Farms when Marcus was still a wee little guy. One of the exhibits was a cow milking demonstration where they would lather up ol' Molly's teats, slap on the "milking cluster" (horns), turn on the unusually loud pump, and relieve her poor sagging self. It was rather amazing, amusing, demoralizing, and far too close to home all at the same time. I could tell my older two were not only captivated by the process; they were also COMPARING it to something they had seen many times before. I just thought I would warn you in case you ever hear the words, "milking demonstration in five minutes" uddered.

Some Habits Die Hard

Breast milk can be a magic weapon when it comes to getting baby some zzzzz's. I have a friend who actually tried to nurse her little guy back to sleep one night a month or so AFTER he was weaned—desperate for some rest and knowing how well it had once worked. (Sadly, it did not help that night.)

Here are three scenarios breastfeeding moms often find themselves up against and some tip-of-the-iceberg advice to fix it (if and when you and your family decide it needs fixing). Please keep in mind as you read this that I am by no means an expert; but I have definitely felt your pain, learned from it, and lived to tell about it.

Nursing Baby to Sleep. Nursing your baby before bed provides a wonderful time to cuddle and bond—especially for breastfeeding moms who work outside the home. It's also nice to fill up the tank so your baby will hopefully sleep a little longer! But there's a big difference between that scenario and what I remember going through to get Lena to sleep at night. I would nurse her and then spend about fifteen minutes transferring her into the crib that was no more than three feet away—putting her down ever-so-delicately, inch-by-inch for fear of waking her during the process. If she woke up at any point, we would begin the process again—nursing, rocking, soothing—the whole shebang. I loved our baby girl, but the bedtime "routine" was getting a bit old.

Of course, it wasn't her fault. She had not learned how to fall asleep on her own because we had never given her the opportunity to try. In fact, it wasn't until she was nearly a year old (after several nights of letting her cry it out) that she finally "learned." We certainly "learned" our lesson the hard way and decided to be more proactive with our other two. I would still nurse them before bed, but that was followed by reading a few books and singing a little song on the way to the crib. They would go to bed drowsy but awake, and that made all the difference.

Have you crossed over from nursing for the bonding experience to nursing so your baby will sleep? As long as you, your spouse, and baby are happy with the arrangement, by all means do it! Just realize that this *can* be habit forming—especially after baby hits the fourth-month mark and beyond. That's when most babies can (not that they *do*, but they *can*) soothe themselves and fall asleep on their own. The longer you wait to break the cycle, the more difficult it may become.

Night feedings will be inevitable for some time. I sure wish I could tell you how long but I can't since every baby and situation is different. According to Weisbluth, breastfed babies *should* be able to sleep through the night without any liquid encouragement by 9 months. Marcus did not get that memo. He went to sleep on his own wonderfully, but he wanted MAMA in the middle of the night on no uncertain terms. In retrospect, I think if I had given him more time to fall back asleep on his own and not gone in so quickly for night feedings, he would have slept through the night much earlier. As it was, he didn't end night feedings until he was practically weaned. I knew he didn't NEED any food in the middle of the night, but his body thought he did because of a habit we had formed. I call it the "I-am-crying-and-need-mommy-to-nurse-me-back-to-sleep" habit. It was a tough nut to crack.

Through several trials and errors, we finally came up with a plan for success. We installed black-out curtains (since his bed faced the road) and also began playing a sound machine in his room. And since babies can smell their mamas from far away, I was evicted to the guest bedroom downstairs where our little bloodhound couldn't sniff out my breast milk. My dear hubby took over and used the Ferber method of going in with increased intervals of time in between each visit to help soothe him back to sleep. It was an emotional, vociferous period of time, but he eventually caught on and now sleeps through the night on a regular basis. It's not for everyone, but it certainly did the trick for us.

Co-sleeping definitely provides the most sleep for the most people. And as long as it works for your family (and it's done in a safe manner), it's not so much a habit as it is a lifestyle. This arrangement may work for months; it may work for years. But at some point, at a mutually-agreed upon time, your child will leave the nest. Obviously the older the child gets, the more difficult the transition may be. I've spoken to some friends about this emotional transition. Some moms said that they would have their child sleep on a mattress (the one that would eventually belong on his crib/big boy bed) next to their bed and gradually (week-by-week) moved it further and further away, then out the door (in the hallway) , then into his bedroom, and eventually into his crib/bed.

Another option is to begin by having them take naps in their bed. After they are accustomed to that, you can get them in their jammies and read books in their bed. Lastly, when the time is right (and let them know it's coming with plenty of positive hype), lay them down in their own bed at night. One friend would tell her little guy that she'd be back in two minutes to sing him a song/soothe him IF he stayed in his bed. When he realized he would be rewarded for his patience, he started staying in bed and she gradually increased the time between visits until he began falling asleep on his own. It was a rocky few weeks, but it eventually worked like a charm.

To Wean, or Not to Wean: That is the Question

Although I ultimately suggest trying to breastfeed for <u>at least</u> a year, my advice is to make your goal AT LEAST seven weeks. Baby will have just finished a major growth spurt (and will subsequently make it longer between feeds), and you'll be heading out of the initial mommy-fog. If you make your goal six weeks or less, you will have missed the reward for all your hard work! Who knows…once you conquer seven weeks, you might be surprised at how much easier it gets and decide to go longer. And moms returning to work can be empowered by the many mothers in this book who went back, and, despite the obstacles and challenges, met or exceeded their breastfeeding goals. Where there's a will, there's a way.

Just promise me that before you throw in the towel (or nursing bra as the case may be), you consult with a lactation consultant, get online, find a pro-nursing group that fits your lifestyle, or find a fellow nursing friend who can lend advice or a shoulder to cry on. Like any other goal in life, breaking your nursing "career" into smaller sections of time (just one more day…just one more week…just one more month) will help significantly. See Kerri's story on page 171, Sherri's story on page 169, and Gwen's story on page 187 for more on goal-setting and how support from family and friends can help.

I remember my high school cross country coach handing out a list of excuses vs. reasons for not running. He must have realized that we just wouldn't feel like it some days—and the same certainly holds true for nursing. I would be lying if I said I loved all 365 days of nursing my three kiddos. There were ebbs and flows just like anything else. That's why I have developed the following information to help you discern legitimate reasons for weaning or supplementing versus excuses. I've also added accompanying solutions to the excuses that may get you back on track.

Reasons to Wean Baby Early. Breast is best, but sometimes despite your best intentions, things don't go as planned. If you find yourself struggling with any of the following challenges (after seeking help to fix them), I'd say it is perfectly valid to wean your baby earlier than expected.

- If baby was born with teeth and already knows how to use her chompers, it may be very painful to continue nursing.

- Consistently poor latch (even after visits to a certified lactation consultant for advice on technique).

- You are pregnant again. Although it can be done, it's still a valid reason to stop nursing earlier than expected. If you choose to continue, keep in mind that your milk will eventually turn back to colostrum near the end of pregnancy.

- You have to go on long-term drugs that may affect baby. Check with your baby's pediatrician and your internist or OB/GYN to fully understand the side effects of the drug(s) you'll be taking. Research the <u>Medications and Mothers' Milk: A Manual of Lactational Pharmacology</u> book by Thomas Hale before you write it off. Also read Deidre's story on page 105 for inspiration to get back on track.

- Baby has cleft lip, micrognathia, or the like. Although it can be done in some circumstances, it will obviously take a great deal of strength, perseverance, and support to overcome.

- Constant pain during breastfeeding due to medical conditions. Ensure you have seen a lactation consultant before weaning for this reason. Sometimes the smallest changes to position can reap great benefits. See Holly's story on page 141 and Catherine's story on page 159 for more on latching. See Amy's story on page 101 for an understanding look at pain during breastfeeding.

- Severe injury to mom.

- You are a mother of multiples. This does not have to be a deterrent, but I can't blame any mom for trying and deciding it was too much. See Rachel's story on page 81.

- Breastfeeding causes such significant and constant stress and/or anxiety that it's affecting you, the baby, and/or family relationships. No good shall come of that. Ensure you've exhausted all your resources and consulted with a lactation consultant or a fellow nursing mom who is like-minded and authentic enough to discuss your breastfeeding struggles with. See Peggy's story on page 75, Jacque's story on page 111, Kerri's story on page 171, Jodie's story on page 207, and Sarah's story on page 217 for encouragement and wisdom.

Excuses for Weaning Baby Early. In addition to the reasons listed above, there are also a handful of breastfeeding challenges you may face that leave you *wanting* to wean earlier than expected. You are not alone in having these feelings and challenges, and hopefully the following table of excuses with accompanying solutions will get you back on track.

Excuses for Weaning Baby Early

Excuses	Solutions
It's too hard.	It IS hard and it's easy to lose perspective when you can't see the light at the end of the tunnel. Try to make small goals...just one more day...one more week...one more month. Splitting it up into smaller steps helps tremendously. See Kerri's story on page 171, Sherri's story on page 169, and Gwen's story on page 187 to gain some perspective and encouragement to keep going.
I don't know anyone else who is breast-feeding, so it's hard to keep going.	Attend a LLL meeting, hop on a forum or website (like Facebook.com/MilkDiaries or others from page 68), or call your lactation consultant/local lactation supply store to find a support group near you. Meetup.com is also a great resource for finding like-minded mamas in your zip code. It may be intimidating at first, but just think...you're joining a group of moms who sought the exact same support you need.
I got mastitis/ thrush.	It IS painful and physically draining to have mastitis, and thrush is no walk in the park. However, it will help purge the sickness if you continue to breastfeed. See Kelly K's story on page 91, Deidre's story on page 105, Holly's story on page 141, and Sarah's story on page 217 for tips and encouragement.

Excuses for Weaning Baby Early (continued)

Excuses	Solutions
I have constant low milk supply/my milk isn't coming in.	Find ways to relax, get plenty of sleep, and drink clear fluids!! Easier said than done, I know. But focusing on the basics will ensure you're doing the best you can for yourself and baby. After that, try pumping to stimulate more milk production and/or purchase some brewer's yeast, fenugreek, or other lactation enhancers. I also just heard about a product called MilkMakers—cookies filled with ingredients to boost your supply. Sure wish I had known about those a few years ago! There's a good book called <u>The Breastfeeding Mother's Guide to Making More Milk</u> by Diana West and Lisa Marasco to help you through this as well. Lastly, remember a lactation consultant or resource center is just a phone call away. See the Let's Get This Party Started section on page 24, Peggy's story on page 75, Rachel's story on page 81, Kelly K's story on page 91, Jacque's story on page 111, Kerri's story on page 171, and K.C.'s story on page 199 for more information and encouragement to help you with this common, yet difficult breastfeeding issues.

Excuses for Weaning Baby Early (continued)

Excuses	Solutions
My baby is tongue tied.	This can be a tough call depending upon the severity; but there are options. See Kelly K's story on page 91, and contact a lactation consultant as well as baby's pediatrician to determine a possible solution.
Social norms	Talk about a sensitive subject. Although the world's average age to wean is 4-5 years, mothers in the *United States* who choose to breastfeed past a year may be met with cutting looks or snide remarks. Insensitive comments like, "if a baby can ask for it, she's too old to nurse," or (my favorite) "if a kid can chew a steak, she's too old to be breastfeeding!" may unfortunately cause a mom to think twice before continuing to nurse. When you choose to wean is YOUR choice and no one else's. "To each her own" is what I always say. You are certainly not alone, and with a few clicks of the mouse you can discover a group of dynamic, like-minded moms. You may like Leslie's story on page 179, Mary Ellen's story on page 161, or Mindy's empowering story on page 221.

Excuses for Weaning Baby Early (continued)

Excuses	Solutions
I'm too tired; baby isn't sleeping.	The first 6-7 weeks of a baby's life can be rather unpredictable. Rest-assured, your baby will eventually learn her days from nights and as she gets older and older, she will sleep for longer periods of time. This will be the most sleep deprived you will be (at least until he can drive)! Seek and accept help; take naps when you can; and consider pumping a bottle so that another family member or a friend can take one of the nightly "feeds" and afford you more rest. See Deidre's story on page 105, Holly's story on page 141, Zoë's story on page 193, the Some Habits Die Hard section on page 40, and the 9 out of 10 Experts Do Not Agree section on page 20 to help you and baby get more rest.
Baby has teeth.	Most babies can be taught not to bite once they learn the "consequences" or have an alternative. See Leslie's story on page 179 or Zoë's story on page 193 for tips to tackle biting and make nursing comfortable again. This Ask Dr. Sears link also offers several options to try with your little chomper: http://www.askdrsears.com/topics/breastfeeding/common-problems/bites-breast.

Excuses for Weaning Baby Early (continued)

Excuses	Solutions
My family is un-supportive.	This can be tricky, and lack of support can manifest itself in many ways. My advice would be to stick to your guns and find support outside of your family. Some family members may be opposed to nursing because it takes them away from baby. If that's the case, be sure to find other ways they can be involved (changing diapers, rocking baby, feeding bottles if baby takes them, etc.).
	Some family members may be unsupportive because society has chosen to sexualize breastfeeding. The worst thing you can do in that situation is to "flaunt" it. You aren't going to win them over or do yourself any favors. My advice would be to remain as modest as possible while still maintaining your decision to breastfeed your baby. If it fits your lifestyle, strike a compromise and allow them to bottle-feed your baby some breast milk. You CAN overcome this obstacle!

All Good Things Must Come to an End. At some point, the nursing relationship is going to end. Some moms allow the baby to decide when nursing is over. Other moms make the move when junior gets teeth! Another group of moms let the calendar decide. The AAP recommends that babies exclusively breastfeed for about the first 6 months of life and the continuation of breastfeeding for 1 year or longer as mutually desired by mother and baby. The World Health Organization (WHO) ups the ante with a recommendation to nurse for two years of age and beyond (closer to other countries' norms). Ultimately it is up to you and your family to decide; no one else can or should make the decision for you.

I, for one, am a calendar girl. As I have mentioned, my goal was to breastfeed my kids for a year, and I reached that "goal" with all three! In fact, I made it a little longer with our little guy, as I wasn't quite ready to pull the plug as fast during my "final chapter."

My plot began months earlier when I introduced them to a sippy cup of breast milk. About three weeks before their birthday, I would begin to ever-so-slightly introduce cow's milk into their sippies (a ¼ cup increase per week) so they would get accustomed to the taste and their tummies would gradually acclimate. It worked like a charm for Lena and Marcus.

It actually didn't work so well for my second born. She could sniff out the imposter cow's milk a mile away! However, our clever connoisseur did like juice. So I would mix part juice, part breast milk, and [eventually] part cow's milk together in a little sippy cocktail instead—progressively increasing the amount of cow's milk and decreasing the amount of breast milk and juice. By her first birthday, she was drinking an entire sippy cup of cow's milk without complaint. Now she drinks about two cups of milk a day and juice about once a week.

Not all Sippies are Created Equal. Most sippy cups have a rather large spout that a baby has to tip up for milk to come out—much like a bottle. My kids never took to that because they were used to the sucking motion from nursing. For that reason, I found that straw cups worked best. Apparently they are better for their dental hygiene because the milk doesn't rest on their teeth and gums. You may notice that some brands market straw cups for an older child (like "Stage 4"). I have not found any medical/safety reasons to support this; instead, consider your child more sophisticated and capable for mastering a straw cup so early!

Your Body

Your Weight. Ah...the JELL-O® belly that a new baby leaves behind. I'm sure you've heard that moms who breastfeed lose weight faster, and I tend to agree. This is two-part: nursing helps contract your uterus so your stomach can return to non-rotund size faster. You are also feeding for two and thus expending more calories (provided you don't eat for three or four).

All of that said, don't feel too badly if it's difficult to shed that last 5-10 pounds of baby love. Your body holds onto some reserves until baby is fully weaned so that in the event you become severely malnourished, you can still feed your baby. Although it's not so great that it means holding onto some unwanted "fat tire" a while longer, it's pretty amazing that your body has this built-in feature in case of an emergency. See Leslie's story on page 179 for more on this sometimes sensitive topic.

Working Out. Cut yourself and your baby some slack by easing back into a workout routine. Take it easy and consult with a physician before going back full throttle. Also remember to drink even MORE clear fluids to ensure you're well hydrated. It can be done! See Susan's story on page 213 for a great success story of juggling a "breastfeeding workout" with an exercise workout.

While we're on the subject of exercise, a friend of mine mentioned that her baby sometimes rejected her milk right after a hard workout because it tasted sour. When you work out, your body releases lactic acid and this can be passed on to baby. Besides the potentially sour taste, there are no harmful side effects. Just pay attention to how your baby reacts (if at all), and adjust the time or exertion level of your workout accordingly.

Your Period. Aunt Flo is bound to come back at some point postpartum, although at least for most there's a delayed return as a result of breastfeeding. The break sure was nice while it lasted, wasn't it? Here are a few things you *may* experience around that time:

- Everyone's body is different, but many of my friends agreed that their period came back around the same time that baby began sleeping through the night (your prolactin levels begin to decrease when you begin to nurse less often). Also, be on the lookout for plugged milk ducts when baby starts sleeping through the night!

- You might experience a lower-than-normal milk supply near the return of your period. There's a major hormonal shift taking place in your body. Drink even more clear fluids to make sure you stay hydrated!

- As your period returns more regularly, you might notice your flow is heavier. Ughh. This is not a result of breastfeeding; it's a result of hormones increasing the lining of your uterine wall. I just thought I'd warn you! P.S. That heaviness may compound with each subsequent kid. Double ughhh. Working out on a regular basis can help. If the heaviness gets out of hand, you can consult your OB/GYN to explore alternatives.

Let's Talk about Sex (or lack thereof). I think larger-than-normal breasts during late pregnancy and postpartum is God's great consolation prize to our husbands, something to bide their interest during the hiatus before "resuming normal activity." I have a friend whose husband actually placed a big star on the calendar the day she could resume such activity. She was stunned; but I guess you can't blame the guy for trying.

Let's be honest…between major sleep deprivation and recently becoming the resident milk production facility, the last thing you really want to do is have sex. And there are some legitimate psychological, mental, and physical reasons that you may feel that way:

- Perhaps only second to the fear you have during that first post-baby bowel movement is the fear of what sex might feel like post-partum. If you had a C-section, will your wound hurt? If you had a vaginal delivery, are your stitches fully healed? It is important to see your OB/GYN before resuming sexual activity for this very reason. He/she can ensure your body has healed properly.

- Finding the energy and time is very difficult.

- Hormones are partly to blame as well. Your body's estrogen levels drop dramatically after baby arrives which will make you feel drier down yonder. Estrogen takes a back seat while prolactin begins to work overtime to help make and maintain your milk supply.

- Your body's "new normal" for some reason just isn't screamin' sexy.

- Your body has been touched enough for one day!

All that being said, and despite his sleep deprivation and having witnessed some of those changes and fluids your lower half has experienced, your husband is probably ready and willing even if you aren't.

So what's a girl to do? The best thing you and your spouse can do is be honest, realistic, and sympathetic to each others' needs. A little compromise and creativity can go a long way.

Also don't be surprised, when you do resume normal activity, if you produce an unexpected milk puddle at the end. Why? Oxytocin is the hormone responsible for milk let-down and it's also released during orgasm. Now you know.

And finally, one last but certainly not least public service announcement: you can get pregnant while nursing! Enough said.

What Goes Up Must Come Down: The Laws of Physics and Boobs. My mom is always so nice about noticing when I seem to be losing weight (and also nice about keeping her mouth shut when I don't). It seemed like when Marcus was weaning that my mom mentioned me losing weight about every time I saw her! Funny since my jeans still felt two sizes too small. I finally pieced it together: although the rest of my body remained the same, my *boobs* were beginning to deflate! Be forewarned that when you are finished nursing, your boobs could quite possibly be smaller and less perky than they were before. *Sag* but true.

I'll Drink to That! I was taken aback when a close friend told me that drinking a bottle of beer would not only help me unwind but could improve my milk supply (because it contains brewer's yeast, a substance known to promote lactation). Was it that blatantly obvious that I needed a drink? Although the milk-making benefits to drinking beer is disputed, I'm not about to dispute the psychological effects.

The AAP states that one alcoholic drink while breastfeeding— the equivalent of a 12-ounce beer, 4-ounce glass of wine, or 1 ounce of hard liquor—should not harm your nursing baby. If you choose to have an alcoholic drink, it's best to do so just after you nurse or express milk rather than before and allow at least two hours per drink before your next breastfeeding or pumping session. That way, your body will have as much time as possible to rid itself of the alcohol before the next feeding and less will reach your baby.

Milk Storage Guidelines

I inadvertently threw out a lot of perfectly good breast milk because I didn't know the storage guidelines. You worked hard to pump that milk, so follow the tips and table below so you don't commit the same mistakes I did:

- You'll want to store your liquid gold in 1-4 ounce individual servings and only thaw out one serving at a time to avoid wasting any milk.

- Always label your container with the date/time, and use the oldest one first.

- Never microwave breast milk—it's best to thaw it in the fridge, but for quicker thawing you can hold the container under increasingly warmer running water.

- To warm breast milk, either place the milk in a container of warm water or use a bottle warmer.

- Do not shake breast milk; it's normal for the fat to settle at the top like that.

- If baby does not finish milk at one feeding, it may be refrigerated and offered at the next feeding before it is discarded.

- Make sure to clean and sterilize your equipment between feedings. Using a microwave sterilizer makes cleanup fast and effective. See more in the next section.

Milk Storage Guidelines

Room Temp	Refrigerator	Self-contained Freezer Unit	Deep Freeze
6-10 hours	3 days (ideal) up to 8 days	3-4 months	6 months (ideal) up to 12 months
66-72° F 19-22° C	32-39° F 0-4° C	0° F -18° C	0° F -18° C
Use at next feeding or discard.	Either transfer to freezer within 7 days; use; or discard.	Once frozen, breast milk may be thawed. Once thawed, it should be used within 24 hours. Do not refreeze breast milk.	
Data for this table courtesy of KellyMom.			

Gear

Like any good expectant mother, I agonized over our registry. What's the best high chair on the market? Should we register for the BOB® jogging stroller or the Baby Trend®? What diaper pail could possibly contain the stench (even if breastfed baby diapers stink way less)?

I'll save you much ado about nothing by highlighting several things you may NEVER need on your registry and follow up with some "musts" or at least "maybes" to consider as a breastfeeding mom.

- ***High Chair.*** We soon exchanged our ginormous (as Anna would call it) high chair for a booster seat. It saves so much room, cleans up easier, and functions just as well if not better than a high chair.

- ***Diaper Pail.*** I would contend that over time no diaper pail on the market can contain the stench well enough, so getting rid of the diaper itself was our preferred option. We started using a normal trash can with a lid to hold diapers and emptied the contents each night or as needed.

- ***Changing Pad Cover.*** Consider using towels on baby's changing pad instead of registering for a fancy cover. They are so much easier to remove, you have plenty in stock, and chances are you have several colors to choose from to match the nursery.

- ***Books.*** Don't register for books about baby's first year and breastfeeding. Purchase and read them now! Reading a variety of books may help you determine the kind of lifestyle you and your family choose.

- ***Lovies.*** This is something I tell every expectant mom I know. Instead of registering for a couple of fancy lovies with animal heads or tags coming out of everywhere, buy about three sets of thin burp cloths (we liked the Gerber® terry burp cloth 3-pack) to keep your baby feeling safe and secure. You can have some in the wash and some on hand, they are lightweight and easy for baby to grasp, AND you'll have plenty of replacements when Jr. decides to throw them out of the shopping cart...or in the trash...or in the sand box just to name a few.

I feel like getting out the registry gun just talking about all of this! Good times. Next let's talk about some great recommendations to make your nursing life a little easier. Also see the Breastfeeding Product Websites section on page 70 for a list of virtual stores that carry the following products:

- *Nursing Pillow.* ~~Buy a Boppy® pillow!~~ Buy **TWO** Boppy® pillows (one for the bedroom and one for the living room; or one for upstairs and one for downstairs; or one for Grandma's and one for...you get the picture). It's always nice to have an extra—or at least an extra cover for the inevitable spilled milk, spit up, or host of other fun bodily functions that may find their way to your Boppy® pillow.

  I heard such good things about the Boppy® pillow before Lena was born that one accompanied us to the hospital. I must admit I had limited success trying to use it there. Maybe it was the orientation of the bed or the 1,000 pillows behind me, but it just didn't work. I'm so glad I gave it another shot once we got home because it sure was a back saver. Later it was the perfect platform for her to have tummy time.

- *Pump up the Volume.* A breast pump is a nursing mother's companion whether you plan to go back to work or stay at home—affording flexibility in your schedule and a degree of separation from baby when necessary.

You may wind up using it much more often than you originally intended. I know I did.

Perhaps the only difficulty in registering for a pump is deciding which type you will need. I originally registered for a hand pump—thinking I would be at home and wouldn't need much more. It served its purpose until (dun, dun, dun) my low milk supply issues began. That's when I borrowed a Pump-In-Style® double breast pump from a friend, and it did wonders for my supply. I was also glad we had it during our move when my parents would watch Lena while we went house-hunting. Think through the lifestyle you intend to have and register/buy accordingly. Medela actually has a nifty product selector available on their website.

If you're unsure about how often you plan to use a pump, consider borrowing/buying a used pump from a trusted friend and simply use replacement tubes, horns, etc. (A lactation supply store should be able to determine what replacement parts you'll need.) Read Sherri's story on page 169 and Zoë's story on page 193 for more about breast pumps. For a good laugh, read Kim's story on page 125.

- *Bras.* I used nursing bras the entire year with my first. I only used them a couple months with my second. I think I burned them before Marcus was born and settled for tank tops instead. My advice would be to buy one or *maybe* two and make sure you like them before buying too many. Also wait until the last month or so of pregnancy to go bra shopping because you're only gonna get BIGGER once junior arrives! Most lactation supply stores not only stock nursing bras; they also offer bra fittings. Read Holly's story on page 141 for more advice about bras and bra fittings.

- **Nursing Pads.** I used Lansinoh® disposable nursing pads to manage leaks and found they worked really well. Of course, other moms may prefer the reusable type. You may need to wait a week or two into nursing to have a better feel for what you need. Your choice may come down to environmental concerns; or it may come down to how much milk you produce (or overproduce). Whichever way you go (disposable or reusable), suffice to say that they come in handy!

- **Topical Cream/Lanolin.** Lanolin rocks! I would rub it on my breasts after every feeding for several months with each baby, and I think it made a big difference. There are several different brands available. I found Lansinoh® to be the easiest to apply.

- **Nursing Cover (aka Hooter Hider).** Blankets never did the trick for me. Either my shoulders would slump and the blanket would fall off or baby would grab a handful and pull it off for me. If you're as uncoordinated as I am, don't fret and don't allow that fear to keep you from eventually and modestly nursing in public. There are quite a few contraptions on the market to make nursing in public more discreet. Several wraps and slings on the market make nursing in public modest and easy as well.

Nursing in public is a learned artform, so begin by practicing at a friend's house and work up your courage to venture out more and more. Most other moms understand and men really don't know what you're doing unless their wives nursed (in which case they are probably used to the scene). Case in point: One night I was nursing Anna at an outdoor concert and chatting with a man in front of me the entire time. He was flabbergasted when, after a good feed, she appeared out from underneath my hooter hider! Just try not to flash anyone purposefully and buy a hooter hider so it's never an issue. See the Breastfeeding is Natural? section on page 29 for more tips for nursing in public and read Mindy's story on page 221 for encouragement.

- *Microwave Sterilizer.* If you plan to pump, that means you plan to clean a LOT of bottles, horns, and other fun contraptions. Do yourself a big favor and buy a BPA-free microwave sterilizer. A friend of mine gave me one as a shower gift, and I had no clue what it was. Once Lena arrived, I realized how much time and energy it saved. It's basically a dome-topped microwavable container that sterilizes all of your bottles and pumping equipment in five minutes flat. No dishwasher; no boiling water; just thoroughly rinse out your equipment, place it in the sterilizer with a bit of water, and nuke for five minutes. Life is good. You could also register or buy a few microwavable bags that work the same way (and may provide a working mom a way to carry her clean pump parts back home). To read more about pumping, bottles, and storage, see Lanee's story on page 163 and Kerri's story on page 171.

- **Bottles.** You may have every intention of exclusively breastfeeding. But experience has taught me to be prepared, and I suggest you do the same by having at least a set of bottles readily available. We had good luck with the Dr. Brown's brand and I liked all the nipple varieties they provided. Medela also has a product on the market called the Calma® that requires babies to mimic the suck motion necessary for breastfeeding.

- **Baby Sling.** I never mastered wearing my sling (I'm rather spatially challenged), but don't let that stop you from trying. It's a wonderful way to bond, swish your baby to sleep, and/or hold your baby while still getting a thing or two accomplished. From the Moby® to the Maya® to the Balboa Baby® wrap, the only trouble is deciding which one to choose!

- **Milk Collection Bags.** You may want to purchase some bags to save any expressed milk. You can also use sandwich bags to hold that liquid gold (see Lanee's story on page 163 and Kerri's story on page 171 for more on that). Also check out the Milk Storage Guidelines section on page 58 to learn more about properly handling and storing breast milk.

Resources

Books

Quite a bit of literature is available on the subject of breastfeeding. If you're looking for more information or inspiration, check out these reads:

- **The Nursing Mother's Companion** by Kathleen Huggins. This book is a comprehensive "how-to" guide (for when things are working as well as when they aren't) with up-to-date medical information and product reviews for expectant and nursing moms.

- **The Complete Book of Breastfeeding** by Sally Wendkos Olds and Laura Marks goes beyond latching techniques and milk supply—providing relevant information on all aspects of having a new baby (like how to get baby to sleep, pumping, going back to work, etc).

- **So That's What They're For** by Janet Tamaro provides a light-hearted, inspirational guide to breastfeeding basics.

- **Nursing Mother, Working Mother** by Gale Pryor and Kathleen Huggins provides valuable tips for moms who want to successfully juggle working and nursing.

- **Spilled Milk** by Andy Steiner offers down-to-earth stories and advice to remind nursing moms they are not alone.

- ***Milk Memos*** by Cate Colburn-Smith and Andrea Serrette was "born" when several moms began a journal of advice and support for each other in IBM's employee lactation room.

- ***Hirkani's Daughters: Women Who Scale Modern Mountains to Combine Breastfeeding and Working*** by Jennifer Hicks was inspired by an ancient Indian tale. It is filled with stories from moms who went back to work and continued to breastfeed.

Helpful Websites

The web certainly does not lack for breastfeeding information. The trick is finding sites that fit your particular nursing lifestyle. Below is a list of some leading breastfeeding sites along with a short description of each.

- ***Ask Dr. Sears*** provides a wealth of information about breastfeeding and other baby topics like nutrition and vaccines. http://www.askdrsears.com

- ***Best for Babes*** seeks to "beat the booby traps® that prevent moms from achieving their personal breastfeeding goals." They provide help to new and expectant moms, working moms, and more. http://www.bestforbabes.org

- ***Breastfeeding.com*** contains a ton of articles on a variety of breastfeeding topics (and more). http://www.breastfeeding.com/breastfeeding.aspx

- ***Breastfeeding Basics*** provides moms with valuable information and encouragement for breastfeeding. http://www.breastfeedingbasics.com

- ***Circle of Moms*** offers mommy "community" blogs, forums, and more on a variety of subjects—including an entire discussion on breastfeeding. http://www.circleofmoms.com/breastfeeding-moms

- ***Human Milk Banking Association of North America*** is a place for moms who need milk or have milk to donate. https://www.hmbana.org

- ***KellyMom*** can help breastfeeding moms through just about anything! http://www.kellymom.com

- ***La Leche Leauge*** provides advice and encouragement; contains information about breastfeeding and the law; and can help you find a LLL meeting location nearest you. They also have a forum that nursing moms can join. http://www.llli.org/resources.html

- ***Lansinoh*** provides products such as lanolin, breast pads, and pumps. It also has a nifty going back to work checklist for working/nursing moms. http://www.lansinoh.com

- *Medela* not only sells supplies but provides valuable breastfeeding information as well as a search for lactation consultants and supplies in your area. http://www.medelabreastfeedingus.com

- *Meetup.com* helps you find like-minded moms in your area. Get out and meet someone! http://www.meetup.com

- *My Breastfeeding Diet* is for women who want to eat healthfully and transition back into the work out world while breastfeeding. http://www.mybreastfeedingdiet.com

- *Womenshealth.gov* has some great information for moms during the nursing journey. http://www.womenshealth.gov/breastfeeding

- *Work and Pump* is a helpful site for moms who plan to continue nursing after going back to work. http://www.workandpump.com

Breastfeeding Product Websites

Need nursing supplies? Check out these sites (quite a few are courtesy of Leslie. You can read more from her on page 179).

- *Breastfeeding Essentials* has an array of breast pumps, accessories, and supplies. It also has an extensive "library" of information about breastfeeding. http://www.breastfeedingessentials.net

- *Glamourmom.com* proves that you can still look and feel glamorous all while breastfeeding your baby. Check out their nursing tanks. http://www.glamourmom.com

- *Medela* has an extensive variety of breast pumps and supplies in addition to valuable breastfeeding information. http://www.medelabreastfeedingus.com

- *Milkmakers* has baked up some cookies that help breastfeeding moms increase their breast milk supply. http://www.milkmakers.com

- *Milk Mommy Milk* sells slings, nursing clothes, and more for organic parents. http://www.milkmommymilk.com

- *Motherwear* is your one-stop shop for nursing clothes. It also boasts an extensive "customer care" section with great breastfeeding links as well as a guide to nursing in public. http://www.motherwear.com

- *Over The Shoulder Baby Holder* is dedicated to baby wearing. http://www.babymain.com/slings

- *Sparrow's Nest Baby* has an array of nursing shirts. http://www.nestmom.com

- *Stylin Mama* sports maternity and nursing clothes, accessories, and Motherlove® lactation remedies. http://www.stylinmomma.com

- **The Natural Baby Catalog** carries nursing clothes, nursing bras, carriers/slings/wraps, and a plethora of other natural alternatives for you and baby.
  http://www.naturalbabyhome.com

- **The Pump Station** carries a ton of nursing supplies, clothing, and advice for nursing moms.
  http://www.pumpstation.com/pumpstation

Stories of

Determination

A firm or fixed intention to achieve a desired end.

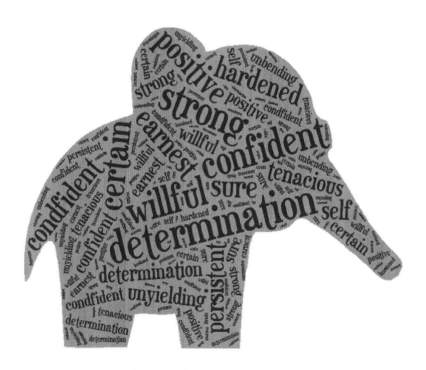

Peggy's Story: Stand by Your Man

I came from a family of nursing mothers. My mom nursed all seven of her children in a time when nursing wasn't very popular. My two sisters and my three sisters-in-law nursed their children. It was all I knew. As far as I was concerned, it was a no-brainer: I would nurse my children as well. I took a nursing class prior to my baby's birth and made sure my husband attended with me. My sister had for years been saying that the number one indicator of a successful nursing experience was a supportive husband. Being the planner that I was, I made every effort to prepare myself and my husband accordingly.

The birth of my first child was not completely what I had expected. I was induced at 39 weeks for hypertension that was brought on by pregnancy. I requested an epidural after the doctor broke my water and in my own little world, labor would progress in a "normal" fashion soon after. I certainly misjudged "normal." I was in labor for 22 hours—including 2 hours of pushing. In the end, I was exhausted! But seeing and holding my son was well worth all the work.

Within 30 minutes, he was at my breast and nursing. Wow! He was a strong sucker. The nurses even commented on his strong suck. I continued to nurse him the length of my hospital stay at regular intervals. At every nursing session, I made sure to have a nurse there to confirm that my son was latched on correctly. By the time we were discharged from the hospital, my milk had not come in yet, but I felt we were well on our way to a successful nursing experience.

The next two days were anything but successful. My milk *still* had not come in and my son was losing a lot of weight. He now weighed 15 percent less than his birth weight of 7 pounds and 10 ounces. The pediatrician was concerned and gave my husband and I detailed instructions for feeding our newborn. Despite our two sleepless nights and my very sore nipples, I was to pump and have my husband give our son all of the colostrum I could muster. Then he should supplement with formula. I was also supposed to attempt nursing him. My pediatrician stressed that we needed to do all three feeding options every 2 hours, and requested another weight check appointment for the following morning.

I was a basket case once we got to the car. My husband dropped us off at home and then went up to Kangaroo Kids, a local breastfeeding supply store, to rent a breast pump. The store also happened to have lactation consultants on staff. Meanwhile, I stayed home with my son and took it all in. As written in my personal journal, "I sat with you and cried. I couldn't believe nursing wasn't going well and I was worried about your weight loss. Dad came home and we did the first attempt at the new feeding routine of nursing—colostrum—and then formula. You inhaled the formula. You were definitely hungry! It took us 1 ½ hours to complete all the steps. We had 30 minutes down time and then we were to start again."

I remember being hooked up to the breast pump and sitting in the rocking chair in the nursery. I listened to the pump do its thing and anxiously awaited a single drop of colostrum in the attached bottle. It was an emotionally painful experience coupled with raging hormones. I remember looking across the hall to where my husband fed my newborn son some of my colostrum from a medicine dropper and then a bottle of formula. The tears flowed rather quickly. This wasn't at all what I envisioned my nursing and bonding experience to be. I felt like a complete failure and I didn't know how to fix it. All I kept thinking was *what was wrong with me?*

To my surprise, my husband had made a lactation appointment for me while he was at Kangaroo Kids. He insisted that I go to the appointment and I knew it was in my baby's best interest. Despite my embarrassment, I went "as commanded." It proved to be a worthwhile appointment. The lactation consultant observed a nursing session and assured me everything would be fine. She told us about some gel packs to put on my cracked and sore nipples. In the end, I was very glad I had gone. I received just the right amount of support and encouragement I needed, coupled with some practical advice.

The next day, we took our son in for a weight check. It was a celebration of sorts that he had gained 2 ounces! The pediatrician recommended a NUK® pacifier and nipple for the bottle and showed us how to squeeze our son's cheeks to make his suck more productive. I was surprised she recommended using a pacifier, but I was open to any suggestions at that point. I was desperate to help my son establish good sucking habits for nursing. We were scheduled for another weight check in three days.

Again, we had another successful weight check appointment. Our son was just 8 ounces from his birth weight at eight days old. He had started nursing from me again and we were no longer using formula because I was able to pump enough breast milk for the bottle feedings. Life was good again and I felt like I had successfully beaten the breastfeeding challenge.

In the end, I nursed my son a complete year. He was a chubby, healthy little boy. I never feared for his weight loss again. In fact, he ended up being in the 90th percentile for his weight once the nursing clicked. My husband rarely gave him bottles because it only took me 7 minutes to nurse him. I could only nurse off of one breast at a feeding because he would throw up everything if I nursed off of both. My milk came down fast, and there was no shortage in volume. I was also able to give him pumped breast milk in public situations with no problem.

The initial hurdle might have scared off anyone, but my sister was right. The number one indicator of a successful nursing experience is a supportive husband. If it weren't for my husband making the lactation appointment, I would have stopped nursing just three days in. I am happy to say that I stuck with nursing and was able to nurse my second son for an entire year as well. That time, I started pumping the minute I got home to bring my milk in more quickly. It was a simple precaution I was willing to take for the benefit of my nursing experience. Looking back on the years I nursed, I smile with pride at our determination to make it work. Our boys had a healthy start to their lives from an emotional and nutritional standpoint. Trying to make it all work was the least I could do.

Rachel's Story: Twice the Blessings

For a year, two months, and fifteen days, I scheduled my entire life around one thing: my breast pump. You see, my twins were born 3 months early—weighing 2 pounds, 7 ounces (Twin A) and 2 pounds, 2 ounces (Twin B)—and pumping was about the only constant during that ever-changing time in my life.

In addition to the twins' much earlier-than-expected arrivals, my husband and three older children would be moving to a new state half the country away just ten days later. That meant I had ten days to recover from emergency surgery; start pumping so that the twins could eat; pack up a house; say goodbye to my husband and other children for at least a month; and then move in with family members and friends for whom I am eternally grateful. To say I was under some stress would be an understatement. Of the century.

Day One

As soon as I was settled in our room after recovery, I requested a breast pump. The one sent in looked more like a medieval torture device than a useful machine to extract milk. What's worse, it *felt* like a medieval torture device, too, pulling at my breasts as if they were made of silly putty! I took a deep breath and started in for ten minutes. Nothing but a drop. Now that was strange because with my other children, I was a cow when it came to milk production! With son number one (who was also a preemie) we joked that I could not only feed the neonatal intensive care unit (NICU) with my surplus—I could feed the entire maternity ward! I exclusively nursed Son Number Two and Daughter as well. In fact, my milk was in with my daughter before we even left the hospital! Breast feeding? Pumping? NO PROBLEM. I'm a pro. . . right?

Day Two

The assistant to my neonatologist came in asked me how I was doing and if I wanted to see the babies. They looked like little baby robins, with lanky arms and legs with no fat on them. Twin A had bruises from the birth process and Twin B was ventilated—not even allowed to move so that the machine could breathe for him. The nurses were kind and helpful, and the twins seemed well cared for, although I must say, emotions were running rampant in my heart and mind.

About that time, a lactation consultant finally came for a visit. I was given a packet of information about pumping with a log to keep track of date, time, and amount (per breast and total expressed). The information seemed to be saying that consistency was the key. So time after time—every three hours—I tried. At lunch, still only a few drops were coming out. Crying, I got myself back into bed. The chills set in and I was alone. My babies were in NICU, my family was busy packing and would be moving soon, and I had no milk.

When my lactation consultant came for a second visit, she had a gift for me: a different pump! In steep contrast to the first model, this pump was nice, neat, and looked like a little boombox on a stand. And because my babies were in the NICU, insurance paid for me to use it! She explained how the pump worked and encouraged me to keep trying—telling me to write down all the progress on the paperwork I was given earlier. It will come, she encouraged. She reminded me that I had been through a lot.

It seemed like *everyone* kept telling me that. *Who cares what I've been through. I am a mother...shouldn't something be coming by now?* Another deep breath and I hooked up (the new and improved) machine with high hopes. But all I got for my efforts was a little colostrum...a couple of drops...that was it. *Are you kidding me?*

I started reading the material—thinking maybe I was missing something that had changed since the last time I did all this. It said to try every two to three hours, ten minutes per side. So that became my new objective. Those first couple of days in the hospital, I would pump, eat, and then walk to the NICU...pump, eat, then walk to the NICU... sleep, pump, eat, and walk to NICU.

Day Three

The day before leaving the hospital, I got really excited! I had pumped enough milk to take an entire bottle to NICU! I couldn't believe it! Three days and five hours after birth, my boys finally had milk from me! This little victory was bittersweet as Twin A would get every drop of this first bottle. Twin B was just too sick to "eat" and had to rely on IVs for his nutrition. I felt a little defeated that all my hard work was partially going to waste, since one of the boys couldn't eat. I just stood looking into the incubators at both my boys.

As I looked at them, I noticed the two nurses who were in the delivery room with the boys. They were doing their work. There were *so* many babies and nurses, and for a moment I felt out of place, like I was in the way and unwanted. I was a mother who could only look and not touch her babies—a woman who stood in the way of the really important people in her babies' lives—those who would be keeping them alive. After a while, I went back to my room and yes, hooked up to the pump because by then it had been two and a half hours since the last attempt. At the time, it was all I could do for them.

Day Four

Heading home as a post natal mother without a baby seems the most unnatural thing in the world. And why is it on the same day, there had to be a "cleaning out" of the maternity ward! Baby here, baby there, I could not escape! Having stuffed everything in the car, we went on our way.

The next few days were filled with the last this and the last that. The last day of school combined with the last day at the park...the last day in our house...the last time we would go to church. All of this was in conjunction with trips to the hospital, packing, and yes—pumping! My goal was to pump every two hours, with maybe every three hours during the night. By the time my family left for our new home, I was getting more than 30 ounces per day! There was finally a surplus!

Goodbye

The morning my family left, we had spent the night at a hotel, and I spent the morning with the children while my husband went around town finishing up some things. We ate lunch together, and then I sent my family off for a two-day trip to our new house. In the car on the way to the hospital after saying good bye, I listened to my good friend's CD and her version of the Doxology. Crying and singing at the top of my lungs, I prayed that God would help sustain me through the next couple of months of not knowing. It was times like these that I was thankful for the two constants in my life: my pump and my faithful log, which by now had an entire page full of milk amounts.

There were times when there were so many babies in NICU that you literally had to find a secret place to pump! I had to pump in the conference room quite a few times and even used the lactation consultants room a few times. Thankfully, everyone there was used to exposed breasts, so while they allowed for your privacy, I didn't feel as if I was intruding on their personal space either. A month in and I was pumping around 50 ounces a day. My babies were growing, but they were not eating as much as I was pumping! They still were unable to suck and ate through a tube!

That's about when disaster struck. Twin B contracted pneumonia. After being off the ventilator for less than 24 hours, he went back on, and on to a stronger machine. Things looked very serious, and it was so hard to keep going. My brother-in-law was getting married that same weekend to boot! My husband and children were flying in and they were involved in the wedding. It was so wonderful to see my older children again, but it was hard because my mind constantly wandered to my sick baby.

Thankfully the wedding did not stop my pumping schedule. I was still able to pump every three hours. There was another woman there who also had to pump, so we bunked up together in the bridal dressing room and talked while the machines hummed in the background. While pumping, the door opened abruptly and a teenage boy walked in—eyeing the champagne and treats on a nearby table. We tried to warn him, but he said he didn't mind and walked right in to find us pumping away. A young kid drinking champagne with two scantily clad women. What an image! Well, I certainly wasn't going to mess up my output numbers for a sixteen-year-old who had no concept of boundaries! He stayed and held a conversation with us while we finished and closed up. And some moms think they've breastfed in some interesting situations!

In those weeks there were many things happening with the twins. I was able to try and feed Twin A with a bottle, and give him a bath. I even held Twin B for the first time (at around six weeks). I also watched babies come in and go home. I enjoyed getting to know other mothers, but my desire to reunite with the rest of my family grew stronger. I felt like I had outstayed my welcome at my in-law's house, and it seemed harder to stay there with no resources. It had been almost two months, and it was time to move on.

We weren't the only ones that made the trip across the country. I also had an entire freezer full of liquid gold! If you ever find yourself needing to ship breast milk halfway across the country, be forewarned that it'll cost you some gold to get it there. First off, it had to stay cold, so I had to pack it all in dry ice. So in addition to all the other errands I ran before leaving, I went to the hardware store—full of big burley men—to get some dry ice. Between the ice and the postage, I spent over $1000 to deliver the liquid gold to my new doorstep. It was worth every penny to fill an entire freezer in the basement!

The twins spent another month or so in the new hospital. Twin B's health improved and all those huge problems seemed to slowly dissipate into smaller things that could be managed with medication. But I had a different life. Still driven by pumping, I not only had to put hospital time into pumping sessions, but now regular wife and mothering work as well. *Do I pump before or after I make lunch? Do I try to put them to bed first, or do I pump first?* Pumping continued to be my number one priority, although it was about this time that I cut back to every four hours instead of three and quit recording everything. I simply had too many things on my plate.

That fall, we settled into a routine of school, dance, gymnastics, swimming, and therapy. Pumping fit into this routine, and nothing could get out of whack because it would mess with the schedule! I would pump at certain times of the day. These times were not to be messed with because it was the food my babies ate. By the time the spring rolled around, I was pumping only three times a day and by the time the twins turned one, I was pumping once in the morning and once at night. My goal was to pump until I had enough milk to last until their (due date) first birthday. In July I had it figured out, and I put my pump away the third week of July with enough milk to last until July 31 for Twin B.

Life after the Pump

What about life after pumping? I look back and I don't know how I did it, especially after coming home from the hospital. It was well worth it, though! I must admit that it was freeing to not be scheduled around the machine any longer, but at the same time, there was a grieving cycle I went through. I would mentally panic that my twins would not get enough to eat, or not have the right kind of food. I also missed the constant in my life.

I spent a lot of time at the beginning of this story on purpose. To those of you mothers with preemie children or with children born who are sick, I hope it is an encouragement to you that there is a way to make it work, if you are interested. I cannot tell you the mothers I have spoken to who wish they would have made a better go at pumping, or at least tried. Just remember to keep up your log and be consistent. At the end of the day, what is most important is that you have a happy baby and you are able to mother that child in the way God allows. Don't stress about it and don't worry. Whatever you get pumped as a new mother is always a blessing to your baby, whether it is a little bit or freezers full! Good luck!

Ann's Story: Dinner Party

I breastfed both of my kids because my mother and grandmother both had breast cancer, and breastfeeding is supposed to help prevent that as well as other illnesses. I was happy to do it for my children and myself. It was a great bonding experience and a very good test of my patience. You see, neither of my children would take a bottle of breast milk, so I was the only supplier of food for them. Unfortunately, I couldn't have help with feedings, get much rest, or give my poor bleeding nipples a break. No one ever tells you that it's going to be hard—even a struggle—to get a child to latch on. There is something very humiliating about having a lactation consultant come up to you, grab your boob, and stick your kid's mouth on it. I'm a very self conscience person and that was really hard for me. However, I don't regret a minute of it. It was an amazing time sitting up in the middle of the night with my little guys. I relished the one-on-one time, having them stare up at me and smile or chomp down on my nipple and laugh in a devilish way while I cried. Who knew an 8-month-old could hurt his mom so much!

I was one of those *lucky* gals who would leak all the time, too. If the neighbor would turn on his lawnmower or a dog would back, I would leak. I remember that I was supposed to go to a party and it was going to be my first night out. I called the lactation consultant to ask her what I could do to stop leaking. I was in tears. She was such a positive person and told me how great it was that I was able to provide *so* much milk for my child. She really put things in perspective. I went to the party with triple the amount of breastfeeding pads in my bra and still leaked! (My friends had a barking dog.) It was horrible and worth it all at the same time.

I think if people told you breastfeeding can be hard, painful, and stressful it would help. I felt like I was the only one who had troubles. If someone told me upfront, I think I wouldn't have stressed about it. I would have just known that it was going to be something I might struggle with. No one wants to feel like they are alone.

Kelly K's Story: The Show Must Go On!

Prior to my first child being born, I wanted to be prepared and feel like I had as much knowledge as I could, because I knew that there would be a lot of "learning on the job." I took a breastfeeding class at the hospital where I was going to deliver, read multiple books, consulted friends, and did online research. No matter how much I prepared, there was no way to apply all of that knowledge without actually having a baby to feed. I was anxious about the process and wanted to feel like I did my "homework" before baby came. Hopefully by sharing some advice I learned "on the job," I can help any moms who may experience some of the same things.

Reagan

I developed thrush soon after my daughter, Reagan, was born. A few weeks before she was born, my doctor put me on an antibiotic because I was very sick and it's possible that was the cause. My pediatrician gave me drops for the baby's mouth, but my OB/GYN gave me an ointment for myself since baby can transfer thrush to the mother. In retrospect, that probably wasn't the best choice to have ointment for myself. Every time I would nurse, I would have to go and wash myself before the baby could nurse because the ointment wasn't something that should be ingested. When I would do this, it would stimulate letdown and I would start dripping like crazy or even squirt. It wasn't a pleasant experience and only caused stress while the baby cried and I was busy cleaning it up. That letdown should have been for the baby! Later, the pediatrician's office told me that I could have put the same medicine I was giving the baby on my nipples. Lesson learned.

Plugged Duct

I had my first plugged duct when Reagan started sleeping for longer stretches at night and another one when she started sleeping through the night. Taking a hot shower with a massage followed by pumping did the trick. Having baby start feeding from the plugged side first helped as well. It is important to keep working with that duct because it can lead to complications if you don't. I also increased some feedings temporarily until the duct was flowing again.

Milk Supply

I had a very good milk supply for the first 4 months. At the beginning, I had such a good supply that my body didn't regulate itself for about a month or two. I went through a LOT of breast pads. I always put a towel down where I was sitting (to save my couch) and put an extra cover on my Boppy® pillow so I didn't have to wash it all of the time!

However, when Reagan starting sleeping through the night, I noticed a decrease in my milk supply. I was very concerned because my goal was to breastfeed her until she was a year old. I exhausted MANY different options and thought it would be helpful to other moms to discuss what I tried and my results.

- I went on fenugreek for several weeks, and later I added Blessed Thistle to my herbal intake. I personally did not find a lot of success with either combination. I used Motherlove's® More Milk Plus for a bit as well, but I didn't find it to be helpful either.

- Along with the herbs, I added more pumping cycles to my day (which ended up making me VERY sore)—including getting back up in the middle of the night to pump. I hated getting up in the middle of the night and it made me feel like a zombie the next day because I was so tired. I felt like I was killing myself to try to increase my supply. After some time, I gave up pumping in the middle of the night because I felt like it was more important to be rested the next day so I could be a more patient, loving mother. (SLEEP!!! It only creates more issues when you don't!)

- I ate oatmeal every day because I heard that it would help stimulate the supply as well. I would even have a beer at night when I had a longer stretch before I would have to feed again to make sure there was no alcohol in my milk. I didn't really find that either of these things worked for me, but it may be great for someone else.

- Lastly I talked to my doctor about taking Reglan to help stimulate my supply. I was a bit hesitant because after doing some research on the drug, the main side effects were exhaustion and depression. I decided that I wanted to give it a try, and in about 3 days, I noticed that my supply was back up and I was back on track. It was a relief to know that my baby was getting enough milk and I didn't have to do all of the extra pumping.

- As time progressed, I found myself becoming more and more tired throughout the day and when Reagan went down for her morning nap, which typically would last 1½ - 2 hours, I would have to nap as well. If for some reason I would have to miss that nap, I was a mess. When Reagan was about 8 months old, I also (finally) admitted that I was depressed. I struggled with the decision to either stick it out until Reagan was a year old, since I was almost there, or get off the Reglan and supplement with formula. I decided to wait until my 9 month appointment with the pediatrician and discuss it with him. Long story short, I decided to stop taking the drug so I could start feeling like a normal human being. It took a couple of weeks, but I soon started feeling like myself again. Looking back, I didn't realize that the drug was affecting me as much as it had. I feel like I lost a little bit of myself during those months and lost some happiness with my baby. I feel like I was doing what was best for my baby nutritionally, but I may not have been as happy as I should have been.

My advice is to be realistic about how drugs can make you feel. Reagan got about half breast milk and half formula the last few months and we were all happier for it. I felt like getting some breast milk was better than none, and my own happiness came back.

The Show Must Go On

I own a dance studio and Reagan was born 5 weeks before the 10th annual recital. My husband and I planned ahead by introducing the bottle at 4½ weeks. This allowed me to run the recital without having to breastfeed—since stopping in the middle of it all really wasn't an option.

Because my body wasn't accustomed to going so long between feedings, I soon found myself "overflowing." While sending a group of 4-year-olds on stage, I noticed the wetness was beginning to run down my stomach.

After asking a coworker to take over for a few minutes, I ran to the bathroom in lightening speed to "freshen up." My dress was soaking wet, but I just cleaned it up the best I could so I could get back to the recital. After all, the show must go on!

Jackson

Things seemed so much easier the second time around. I hardly got sore, and I also was able to recognize what a good latch felt like and how to combat random situations. I went into it with much more confidence and didn't have to worry about the baby getting enough because I knew how to monitor weight, poops, and pees. But I still managed to encounter unchartered territory.

Tongue Tied?

After my son was home from the hospital, I noticed some feeding issues and that his latch wasn't as deep as it should be. During one of his crying episodes, I noticed that Jackson was mildly tongue tied. My husband has a fairly severe case and I knew it was hereditary. So I called my pediatrician's office to discuss the situation and they were prepared to clip the tongue (which made me a nervous wreck to even think about that being done to my little baby). It's actually a very simple, common, painless procedure; I was super anxious for him nonetheless. After going in the office to have the doctor look at it more closely, he advised me not to have the procedure done after all. He said it was such a mild case that the risks outweighed the benefits. His weight gain was good, so he was getting the nutrition that he needed. After time, he was fine, and I got over the tongue tie—although seeing that little thing under his tongue still made me a little crazy. (See more about tongue tie in the Glossary on page 227.)

Plugged Ducts Take 2

With Jackson I found that my left side kept getting sore, and I experienced 3 or 4 plugged ducts. I was able to release the plugs fairly quickly and since it was only one side, I would start every feeding on that side to be sure that it was emptied out every time. After the last plugged duct, I noticed that my supply on that side decreased. It was almost like that side was a bit "defective" if you will. It never did recover, and that side produced about 1-1½ ounces less than my other side. I advise moms to stay on top of things like that and make sure after a feeding that milk is pumped out and frozen as much as time allows for them.

I also suggest to all breastfeeding moms to start pumping sooner than later and work on your frozen supply. That way if your supply should start to decrease or you choose to stop nursing, you still can continue to give your child the nutrition from breast milk for a while longer.

Milk Supply Take 2

I was very concerned that I would lose my milk supply early like I did with Reagan, so I started pumping and bagging milk after feedings a few days after Jackson was born. I wanted to increase my freezer supply so I could dip into that if needed. I had a great supply until about month 4 again. I was very emotional and it made me crazy that I couldn't give my son as much as he needed. I didn't understand why my body did this at the same time as before.

When I noticed the drop, I tried to find time to pump more to increase supply, but I didn't have much luck. I also tried More Milk Plus again, but after going through one bottle I found it only helped a little. I wasn't able to keep up with his needs, and I started dipping into my frozen supply.

I spoke to my lactation consultant about my concerns and she actually reminded me of all the problems I had with Reagan. She told me about a drug called Domperidone (Motilium^{TM}), which [at the time of publication], is not United States Food and Drug Administration (FDA)-approved, but has been known to help moms in Canada and Europe with lactation. I did quite a bit of research on it and discussed it with my OB/GYN and nurse practitioner. We collectively decided to give it a try. The tricky part is that the drug can't be found in the U.S. and I had to get it from Canada through an online pharmacy.

After about 3 days of using the drug, I noticed my supply was up quite a bit; however, I also got random headaches from it. I would take the drug for 2-3 week stretches and then go off it and dip into my frozen supply. By month 9 or 10, I decided to stay on the drug but decrease the dosage, which seemed to work fine. I was able to breastfeed Jackson for the entire year and use my frozen supply when needed. I even had enough frozen milk to easily transition to whole milk.

Weaning

I don't really remember engorgement being an issue when it was time to wean Reagan. With Jackson, I certainly did. My boobs were very sore and felt hard and uncomfortable for about two weeks. A hot shower and a little hand expressing without allowing letdown seemed to do the trick for the times when I was hurting badly.

Gear

One day while I was in the OB/GYN's office while pregnant with Jackson, I was paging through a pregnancy magazine and ran across a product called "Milkies." It is basically a soft plastic thing that catches the letdown from the side that baby isn't nursing on. It holds up to 2 ounces of milk and I find that it saved so much milk for me. I highly recommend it. I used it with every feeding at the beginning; as my milk regulated, I started using it only at the first feeding of the day.

I never used a nursing bra. I hated them. I used my sports bras and still do. I found nursing bras to be cumbersome, and I tell all new moms that sports bras can work just fine. Perhaps they would be more helpful to working moms that need them, but I found that the breast pads and a good supportive sports bra did the trick.

Gotta Love Hormones

With my first child I never had a period. I thought that was what happened as long as one breastfed. With my second child, I actually had light periods randomly and even menstrual cramping quite a bit. I think that when I started struggling with my milk, my hormones were going a bit crazy and my body was having a hard time figuring out what it wanted to do. Just make sure you're prepared with items in your purse or diaper bag in case something comes up unexpectedly. Gotta love hormones!

In Closing

Breastfeeding is a wonderful gift that you can give your child; however, it is NOT an easy thing, at least not for me. I certainly had my highs and lows. I have come to respect that breastfeeding isn't for everyone, and that's ok. I totally respect the moms who do it for a steady length of time and overcome the obstacles that come along with it. Breastfeeding my two kids and reaching my goal of nursing them for a year each gave me a deep sense of accomplishment. Although there were times I wanted to stop early, I'm glad we hung in there!

Amy's Story: The Long and Very Difficult Road to Nursing

When I had my first little boy, I was SO very excited to nurse and be close to him. Much to my dismay, things did not go well to say the least. It wasn't Noah's fault. He latched on like a pro. I, on the other hand, thought I was going to DIE!! I was on a first name basis with my lactation consultant. The whole staff was wonderful with trying to help me. It took three months of meetings and solid pumping before we figured out what exactly was going on.

I tried everything: the shields, cream, guards...no matter what I did, I felt like I was being stuck in the nipples constantly with multiple needles (yes, even when not pumping). Forget about sneezing, coughing, or even my shirt brushing against my nipples. I would go through the roof! Pumping hurt, but not nearly as much as Noah's tongue rubbing on my nipple as he tried to eat. Many times I would sit, pump, and cry. The lactation consultant really was amazed that I continued on. I'm not sure it was the best choice, but I am SO stubborn I was not about to give up.

So, anyway, during one of my many meetings with the consultant, she watched me pump. My nipples turned purple! That was when we figured out I had something called nipple vasospasms. Once we figured that out, the doctor put me on a drug called Nifedipine. It took a little while for it to kick in, but once it did, Noah and I were on our way. I could finally manage the pain and went on to nurse Noah for a year and three months. It was wonderful, but I had to wear a bra the whole time and nothing could touch my breasts except for Noah and only while nursing. But I really did love it.

When I had my second little boy, we knew I would probably have the same problem. So as soon as I had him, I got on Nifedipine. I knew it would take a couple of weeks before it would start working and that I would be pumping until that time. This time I was prepared! The pain started and so did the constant pumping. I never had a great supply of milk, so I really did have to pump as much as I possibly could. Well, two weeks after I had Caleb, I was ready to give on-the-breast nursing a try. I maybe nursed him on the breast a couple of times when, to me, the unthinkable happened. Off to the emergency room with hives. Yes, I became allergic to Nifedipine! I tried taking the pill again just to be sure it was that. Probably not the best choice. The hives were MUCH worse, and I had to stop taking it.

The world crumbled around me. Like I said before, I don't like to give up. I felt like such a failure as a mom. Buying formula was unheard of for me. So I decided to pump again. Back to crying and pumping and having constant stabbing pain in my nipples. It hurt so badly that I had to push Noah away and could not hold him. It was at that point I decided, with much pain and guilt, to quit pumping and go with formula. Not just any formula either…oh no. Caleb required the most expensive formula because he had reflux. Good times all around our house. I always wanted to explain why I was buying formula and not nursing. I felt like less of a woman and mom and judged by others who didn't know what I went through.

So what do you think I did the third time around?! Yes, I tried to nurse and did so for most of one day. By the evening of Elijah's birth, I was in tears and in SO much pain that I decided right then and there that enough was enough. I could not push my babies away because I was too proud to give up. I wish I still did not have those feelings of failure, guilt, and judgment though.

We as moms do the best we can. Some can nurse and some cannot, for whatever reason. I share this story in hopes that you don't beat yourself up like I did. All three of my boys are healthy and happy…one breastfed and two formula fed.

Most importantly, just enjoy feeding your precious little baby by bottle or by breast. It's a special sweet time with them.

Deidre's Story:
The Silver Lining

My beautiful baby boy, our third child, arrived in April. He was a plump, healthy nurser. All was well at the time of delivery...except for me. Apparently my placenta did not spontaneously deliver, so it had to be manually removed (as in the doctor had to literally go in after it and pull it out). I began passing large clots even before leaving the hospital. But rather than boring you with the gory details, I'll move on to my story...

In early May, my uterus was ruptured and my bowel damaged during a dilation and curettage (D&C) to remove the still-remaining placenta. I did not realize that something was still very wrong until hours after returning home. That same night, we returned to the emergency room where I had emergency 5-hour surgery and was then hospitalized. I was faced with multiple complications either from the condition or the surgery as the hours and days passed. I would ultimately remain hospitalized for 7 days.

All the while, I have a 4-week old nursing baby at home! Questions raced through my mind...

How would his grandparents feed him? Would he take a bottle? Would he ever nurse again?

Thank goodness, he took right to the bottle. I had not pumped any milk as he was so young, so it was straight to the formula for him. God certainly kept His loving hand over this tiny new life while I remained hospitalized.

I was 100% convinced that I still wanted to nurse this baby. I had nursed both of his sisters until they were nearly 1-year old. I would have been absolutely devastated if I couldn't nurse him—especially knowing in the back of my mind that this would probably be my last baby. I just knew I had to give it the old college try. So I began, shortly after the surgery, pumping breast milk in the hospital. It was really rough at first. I had been cut open (not like a modern C-section, but rather from the navel down to the pubic bone); I was stapled vertically up the middle; and pumping was downright uncomfortable. Then, as the days passed on and new complications/challenges presented themselves, I became very sick and was moved to the intensive care unit. All the while, we continued pumping faithfully every 4-6 hours, only to see this precious "gold" be mostly discarded. (Due to the multiple medications flowing through my body, the majority of the pumped milk could not be given to baby.)

At this point in my story, that I must give credit where credit is due. The ONLY reason that I was able to successfully pump breast milk for a solid week after major abdominal surgery, while hospitalized, can be attributed to my very dear husband. He would prepare the pump and all its parts/pieces each and every time. He would accurately label the few bottles of milk that could be kept and transport them to the refrigerator at the nursing station. Multiple times throughout the course of this terribly awful week, I was simply too sick or too tired to feel like pumping. It was then that he would do it *himself*...as in literally hold the pump to my body and pump out the milk. I can even remember thinking, *Just forget it. He (our son) is never going to take me back anyway. I don't feel like pumping for the one hundredth time. Just give it up.*

He continued nonetheless. And although my counterpart probably had ulterior motives (like knowing it could cost a small fortune if we had to formula feed our son) in my heart I know he also realized how very important it was to me. He had witnessed the breastfeeding bond and other positive outcomes with our two daughters and wanted this God-given benefit for our son, too.

On the seventh day, I finally returned home. I had spoken with a lactation consultant before leaving the hospital in an attempt to get any and all advice I could in regards to successfully returning my son to the breast. I was extremely nervous that I would get home and he would absolutely refuse to nurse. After all, he'd been on formula in the bottle for a week now! Well, once again, God showed his loving presence to us; the baby latched on IMMEDIATELY. It was as if I had just fed him a few hours before. Never was there even a moment of hesitation. He went from breast, to bottle, and back to breast, all before ever reaching the 6-week-old mark!

Thank you, sweet Jesus, dear husband, dear child of mine, and all of my family and friends who helped us through this setback. I still appreciate all of their hearts and loving support and prayers. Now I can gleefully say that, although this was the worst week of my entire life and I am now unable to carry another child in my womb, I successfully breastfed all three of our beautiful and precious children! This mere fact, my friends, has got to be the "silver lining!"

A Cute Anecdote

My girls still call my "boobs" my "milks." If they happen to see me shirtless, they still make a comment about my "milks."

Mastitis

I can also add that I suffered mastitis once. It was horrendous. It is by continuing to nurse that it got better. As hard as it is and as terribly bad as that latch on hurts, it is the best way to get through it. Whatever you do, don't stop nursing! I would grit my teeth and squeeze something really hard each time the baby would latch on, because it truly hurt so bad. But once she was on and nursing, it wasn't nearly as bad and I knew it was the quickest way to get over it.

Working Mama

YOU CAN successfully nurse while working full time. I did it with my first and I worked full time as a supervisor in the post-closing department of a large mortgage firm at the time. The pumping 2-3 times FAITHFULLY every day actually made me feel close to my baby during the day while we were separated. I would spend each 20-minute pumping session just gazing at her photo I put inside my lovely Pump in Style® backpack. Sometimes I would phone my in-home sitter just to see how she was doing. As you can tell, I MISSED HER DEARLY and decided not to return to corporate America after baby #2 arrived just nineteen short months later.

The relaxation that pumping brought was always just what I needed in the midst of my crazy, busy day. Even when it was really hard to break away to pump, I was always so relieved and refreshed that I did just that. There is book entitled <u>Nursing Mother, Working Mother</u> by Gale Pryor that I highly recommend for those who intend to work and breastfeed.

Jacque's Story: Minor Details

After my baby was born, it took quite a few days for my milk to come in. It took so long, in fact, that I began to wonder if I was going to get any milk at all! My baby had borderline jaundice and they kept telling me that in order to clear up jaundice, he would have to poop it out. I was afraid he wasn't getting enough to eat, so my husband and I made the decision to give him formula just for a few days until the jaundice cleared up. To this day, I think that was the best decision for our situation. I would pump every feeding, take whatever I could get, pour it into the tiny bottle of formula, and feed him the bottle.

After pumping for several days, my milk finally came in! I had boobs like Pamela Anderson! And once my milk started coming in, it didn't stop! I was pumping several times a day in order to empty myself, on top of the regular feedings. I was storing up tons of milk in my freezer, and my little guy even started to have some tummy problems due to my overabundance of milk. He wasn't getting any hind milk, which was making it harder for his tummy to digest. After doing some research, I self-diagnosed myself as having hyper-lactation. I decided to make the change to nursing on one side at a time so he could fully empty that breast—getting the hind milk he needed. It did wonders!

Going Back to Work

Fast forward 8 weeks to when I went back to work. Suddenly I was going from 5:00 AM to 11:30 PM on a mere 4 hours of sleep, working a full day, and then taking care of baby in the evenings. I was living off caffeine and not taking care of myself. That's when my milk supply started to decrease. It was quite a change coming from someone who had too much milk in the beginning. I went on a campaign to increase my milk supply. I started taking fenugreek three times a day, drinking lots of water, and watching what I ate. That was when I made the switch to nurse on both sides each feeding and pumping both sides each time I pumped. My milk supply went up drastically within about four days. Fenugreek was my friend!!! I recommend each and every breastfeeding mother with low milk supply consider fenugreek. It is a miracle herb!

Clog!

I was pumping one day at work and afterwards realized my left breast still felt really full. At first I thought maybe I hadn't had a letdown considering I had barely gotten what I normally pumped out. At the next pump session, I was determined to relax, have a letdown, and get some relief. I sat and looked at pictures of my baby and focused on my breathing, hoping it would help. Nothing. That was when I realized it was something more. It didn't take me long to figure out that I had a clogged milk duct. Within minutes I had texts and emails out to my breastfeeding friends.

"HELP! How do I get this out before my boob explodes?!" I typed frenetically.

Their replies to try "a hot showers, massage, cabbage leaves, and relaxation" came fast but to no avail. *Great,* I thought, *all things I can't do very easily while I'm at work.* At the end of the day, when I finally got home, I took a shower and tried to massage it out. Nothing. Finally, out of desperation, I decided to try something I had read: dangle feeding. I ordered my husband not to come in the bedroom, laid baby boy on the bed, and got on all fours to feed him. Within minutes, I had relief! Whew! I thought I was in the clear. That is until just two days later when the same duct got clogged again. It was a Sunday, so I was home with baby, and immediately tried the dangle feeding—just sure that I would get the same instant relief. Nothing. My poor baby was so hungry each feeding and was getting so frustrated that he wasn't getting milk instantly. After hours of searching on the Internet, more calls/texts/emails to my support group, and lots of uncomfortable feedings, I finally filled a water bottle full of HOT water, rolled it down my breast like a rolling pin, and got some relief. Oh, and I forgot one *minor* detail…in a moment of complete despair, I forced my poor husband to try to suck on my breast so I could finally get relief!!! Oh, to be a fly on the wall in my house that day!! Good times. Thank God I have been clog free ever since!

Famous Last Words

Breastfeeding has been the best thing I have done for me and my baby. Being a working mom, I miss so much of his daily life. There is no greater way to connect with him at the end of the day than to nurse. I joke now that I will nurse him until he is 18 since it's the only time that I get with him that I don't have to share with anyone.

I do wish someone had told me how HARD it was going to be. How frustrating it would be. And how tired I would be! If you are bottle-feeding, daddy (or another family member) can take a feeding. But when you are breastfeeding, nobody else can fill in for a feeding. If you start skipping feedings, you lose your supply! (How come nobody told me that?) Breastfeeding is not necessarily more convenient. You'd think it would be considering you take your boobs everywhere you go, but it's not. My life revolves around feedings, and even when I'm away from my baby, my life revolves around pumping. But it is the best thing I've done for my baby so far. It has given me such a connection with him and created such a bond. I look back now, four months later, and think about those first few days, or even weeks, when my nipples were sore and bloody, my back was hurting from hunching over trying to get him to latch on, and I am so thankful I stuck it out. The benefits are endless.

Stories of Humor

The mental faculty of discovering, expressing, or appreciating the ludicrous or absurdly incongruous.

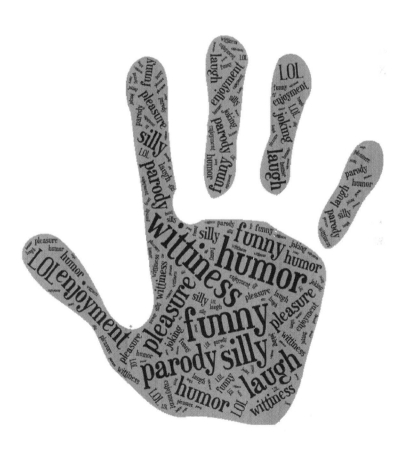

Kelly S' Story: The Lactation Consultant from the Black Lagoon

There is nothing quite like breastfeeding to make a new mom feel like a complete failure at the most important job she will ever have. Scratch that. There is something else: a lactation consultant.

Now before anyone objects, let me say I am perfectly aware that nurturing and helpful lactation consultants exist and are likely the norm. I was lucky to have a good one after the birth of my first child. Unfortunately, despite all the help and understanding she provided, I struggled with little success to breastfeed my daughter. After latching problems, unsuccessful pumping sessions, a painful bout of thrush, and many tears, I gave up after a month. And man, did I feel the guilt. Hence my statement, "There is nothing quite like breastfeeding to make a new mom feel like a complete failure at the most important job she will ever have." But guess what? It turned out okay. My daughter thrived on formula, was happy and healthy, and we both enjoyed feeding time once the stress was gone. That was my first lesson: despite good intentions and all the support in the world, sometimes breastfeeding just does not work out. And that is okay; do not let anyone make you feel otherwise.

This "mommy enlightenment" came in handy when the time arrived for us to welcome our second child into the world. I approached the whole breastfeeding thing much more relaxed. My first choice was to breastfeed, and I went in with that intention. But I knew that if I encountered similar problems to those I had before, I was not going to beat myself up about it. That would not have been healthy for me or my baby. I had this mommy thing down now. No one was going to shake my confidence in my ability and decisions this time around. That was until I met…dun, dun, dun…The Lactation Consultant from the Black Lagoon. We'll just call her Cruella for short.

There I was in the hospital, glowing after the birth of my beautiful, healthy son. Life could not have been better. He was actually doing pretty well with breastfeeding at first, but then he started having some problems latching. No big deal. *I'll just ask for one of those kind lactation consultants to come and give me some pointers*, I thought. It had been three years since I had done this after all. Little did I know what would transpire from this simple, well-intentioned request.

Let me paint the scene for you. My 80-year-old grandmother had just arrived with my aunt to see her new great-grandchild for the first time. We were chatting cheerfully about how adorable my son was and how he had such a perfect little head since he was a C-section baby (take note of that for later). Enter Cruella. She sat herself down right in the middle of our little circle, and I began to tell her the issues I was having. She listened quietly, looked at my chart and said (a little snidely), "You had a scheduled C-section, huh? Well, that's your problem. Your child doesn't know that he is born yet."

[Crickets chirping]...*WHAT????* My blank expression must have said it all. She went on to explain, "You can't take a baby out of the womb before he's ready to be born and expect him to be alert." And there was this *tone* in her voice. I could not believe what this woman was saying to me. I started to get the feeling that she was blaming me for having a C-section, which, by the way, was necessary because my son was breech. Not only that, but she was saying all of this in front of my grandmother and my aunt. How embarrassing. How incredibly embarrassing.

After trying to process what she had just said, I think I stammered out something along the lines of, "Okay, well, I can't un–C-section him, so what do you suggest I do?" Her response: "You have to convince him he's born."

This ought to be good.

She went on to explain that I should not have him swaddled; he should be lying skin-to-skin on my bare chest at all times. Before I knew it, according to her, he would just wriggle his way down to my breast and begin feeding with no problems.

"So you're saying I should be naked pretty much all the time?" I questioned skeptically.

"Yes." And looking right at my grandmother, she added, "So that might mean visitors will have to take a back seat until this little guy gets things figured out." I had never wanted to say, "Oh no she didn't!" more in my entire life.

Now let me interject here that, despite the obvious bitter tone in this retelling, I do understand that Cruella had some valid points. I understand the *idea* behind a scheduled C-section baby "not knowing he's born." I get it. I was not in labor, so technically, the little guy was not ready to come out. And I also understand that skin-to-skin contact is soothing for a newborn. What mother doesn't love snuggling her baby up to her bare chest and feeling that bond? My bitterness comes from how this woman made me *FEEL* in the way she chose to deliver this advice. She had the nerve to come in at one of my happiest times and make me feel like I had done something wrong as a mother. Hence my statement at the beginning of this story. One of the beauties of becoming a mother for a second time is that you can go into the experience feeling confident because you have done it before. So much for that. I had apparently wronged my child right from the moment of his birth, or so she made me feel. And to top it off, she made my grandmother feel as if she was unwelcome to celebrate her new great-grandson. I was livid.

I wish the story ended there, but it doesn't. As she got up to go, she told me that she had a meeting until 3:00 but she would come and check up on me again after that. Oh no. Cruella round two? I thought to myself, *if my son is still not eating by 3:00, she will probably make us reenact the entire birth to help "convince him he is born."* At least I had a couple hours to think of how to get out of this.

Then a glorious thing happened while a good friend was visiting with her young daughter (Gasp! Visitors? Busted.). At around 2:30, my beautiful son performed his first concrete act of love for his mother: he began breastfeeding like a champ! I was so happy, not only because he was eating, but also because at the time he was swaddled up all snuggly and warm, and I was not naked. It was just the opposite of Cruella's advice. I felt vindicated as a mother. My husband, knowing how much I was dreading the second coming of Cruella, suggested that since she would still be in her meeting, I should call and leave a message telling her everything was fine now and that a second visit would be completely unnecessary.

As the phone was ringing, I was planning out carefully what I would say. My thoughts were interrupted by the simple, terrifying word, "Hello?" Oh crap. She answered. I quickly spouted out that my son had begun eating and I appreciated her help. Just as I got ready to say that she did not need to come back, she interrupted, "He's eating right now? Great. I'll be right there." God, why have you forsaken me?

Not two minutes later, Cruella whisked into the room as I sat there feeding my son. Flustered and panicky she clamored, "Skin-to-skin! Skin-to-skin!" At the same time, she scooped up my son, unlatching him in the process, loosened his swaddle, ripped my gown down to expose my chest (in front of my friend, mind you), and tried to get him to latch back on. By now, my son was screaming; he would not latch; my breasts were hanging out there in the breeze; and my friend was in the corner "playing" with her daughter trying to pretend she had not just witnessed this whole thing. If it had not been so absurdly funny, I probably would have cried.

Thankfully, that was my last dealing with Cruella. We brought my son home a few days later, and ironically enough, I had great success breastfeeding him. I made it six months—stopping when he decided that my breasts were great teething toys for his little chompers. It was the complete opposite of what I had experienced breastfeeding my daughter. I had all the wonderful lactation support in the world with her, but could not make it work. And in spite of a total lack of helpful lactation support with my son, I had a wonderful six months breastfeeding him. What is the moral of this story? Well, there are a couple:

First, I learned that the breastfeeding experience with one child does not predict the experience with another child. I am glad I did not let my problems the first time around keep me from trying the second time. But I have also gained the wisdom of hindsight to know that one way was not better than the other. I bonded with my daughter just as intensely and she thrived just as well. I believe that it is not the *method* so much as it is the *mother*.

Which brings me to my second moral: trust yourself and know that you are enough for your child. I learned this when I was able to get over my guilt of feeding formula to my daughter. And I learned it even more so when I realized that the only way Cruella the Lactation Consultant could make me feel like a failure was if I let her. Looking back on the experience, her words do not hurt me. If anything, her words humor me now. I have told this story to many friends and fellow moms who find the experience equally horrifying and hysterical. I laugh at it now because I know in the end, *I* was the one who ultimately knew what would work for my son. Because I am his MOM. And that trumps everything.

P.S. In case anyone is wondering, my son is now four and fully aware that he was born.

Kim's Story: Got Lunch?

I was fortunate to be able to work part time after the birth of my first child. Initially, I went into the office once a week, later coming in more or less frequently as deadlines dictated. I often enjoyed the water cooler talk with co-workers, especially since making the transition from full-time employee to full-time mom and "sometimes" employee was quite an adjustment for me.

As a nursing mom who spent most of my time at home, I did not feel the need to purchase one of the high-end breast pumps. I had the basic model. The case was discreet (plain black) and resembled a large, insulated, soft-sided lunch bag.

As I spent my lunch hour sitting on the toilet, pumping in the one-stall women's bathroom, I often wondered what my co-workers thought of the humming coming from the restroom and the amount of time I spent in there. Luckily most of the co-workers that worked in my building were retired military men. Although I am sure many of their wives nursed at some point and maybe even used a breast pump, I was certain that they were unaware of what was happening in there, and, thankfully, I never had to explain myself.

My point was proven when, one morning, I walked in with the black case carrying my pump and another bag carrying my lunch. I placed the case on my desk and walked to the refrigerator to store my food. As I was returning from the break room, I ran into my co-worker...we'll call him Chester. Chester was a family man, very friendly, and enjoyed finding out what was going on with me when I visited the office. As we chatted, he commented that I must be really hungry, based on the size of my lunch bag. Of course, I knew he was referring to the bag containing my breast pump, but wanting to avoid a conversation about the subject, I simply smiled and tried to steer him to discuss something else.

As we continued to talk, Chester brought up the "lunch" bag again. Again, I agreed with him, "Yeah, I sure am hungry today." On to other topics...*please.*

The third time Chester brought up my hearty appetite, I had had enough. Let's blame it on sensitivity regarding weight gain, hormones, and/or lack of sleep. I practically yelled, *"IT'S A BREAST PUMP...OK?!?!"*

I watched Chester's eyes grow wide in surprise and then realization. Then he stunned me with this winner of a follow-up question, "Oh...so...how often do you have to pump your breasts?"

Really? And I thought it couldn't get any more awkward.

Julie's Story: Poster Child

When I was pregnant with my son, Luke, I wasn't all that passionate and a little on the fence about breastfeeding, but I thought I would give it a try. I was talking with a co-worker who mentioned she used to be a lactation consultant and would be glad to personally tutor me in the breastfeeding preparation class. I was happy for the help and we set a time to get together. I had no idea what was involved in the preparation class, so agreeing to conduct it at our place of employment didn't really phase me. We worked at a local upscale health club, and my friend thought it would be perfectly fine to conduct my "private" class in the aerobics room.

Upon entering our "classroom," she proceeded to pull out these giant posters of breasts and babies latching on—spreading them out over nearly a third of the aerobics room. As she was conducting the class, several 60-something men would come in to do part of their workout—jump rope, lift weights, whatever. They would catch a glimpse of the posters and look completely perplexed and eventually leave. (Obviously my coworker was a lot more comfortable with the topic than I was, as she didn't even flinch when the men entered the room.) I finally just started laughing out loud as my friend, unfazed, finished the "private" class.

The class must have helped to some degree. I went on to semi-successfully nurse my son for six months. I'll never forget our humorous beginnings.

Julia's Story: My Three Sons

A Meal to Remember

Joshua was an early March baby, and we had lots of excitement surrounding our first born. Visitors brought meals and my sister, Tracy, even flew in from Hawaii to meet her new nephew. She was laden not only with luggage; she came bearing gifts as well—namely a beautiful crocheted blanket that matched Joshua's nursery. Gorgeous blues, corals, and hints of fuschia peeked out from the handmade quilt.

Tracy, Joshua, and I had the afternoon to ourselves and decided on an old-fashioned diner for a bite to eat. We had the bright idea of using the new crocheted blanket as a cover up for Joshua's snack. Let's just say it was easier said than done. Pretty soon my sister and I were laughing at my red face as I tried to nurse a new baby in a restaurant, on a warm day, by a sun-flooded window, trying to eat hot food all while feeding a baby under the warm, snuggly blanket! I was flushed; Joshua was squirming; and I was certain I would flash someone!

Well, we made it through our "bite to eat" with lots of warm fuzzies and fond memories to go along with it. To this day, Tracy and I laugh about our special trip to the diner. Joshua is now eight. Some things are never forgotten!

Revelations Happen at any Age

Jared was smaller than my other boys from the beginning. And he never gained much weight despite my nursing him every couple of hours around the clock. At 16 months he was very underweight (13.5 pounds), and we discovered he had severe silent reflux (he had never spit up past 3 months old).

I could hardly keep up with his demands. I was exhausted and hurt from co-sleeping with him in a side-lying position so he could have easy access to my milk. I co-slept with all my children, but Jared was the hardest because he was the smallest and was in our bed the most. Despite my initial fears of him being smothered, I reasoned that I could get more sleep this way.

There were certainly some funny moments sprinkled in with the struggles, though. When Jared was about 6 months old, we set off for a family reunion. I was with everyone in the common area of the house when my husband's uncle shared his brilliant revelation, "She's drinking and he's nursing! They're both drinking!" This was particularly funny to me because he is no stranger to nursing. To my knowledge, all six of his children were nursed! So, I guess revelations can happen at any age!

I Want that Milk too, MaMaMoo!

Elijah, my youngest, was nursed the longest—2 years and 2 months. But long before he reached that age, he'd play this game that is (in my maternal opinion) a sign of his strong will, opinionated voice, and (as the third child) his precociousness.

Every night I'd pump the side that Elijah wasn't nursing on. And every night he'd protest by trying to get his little hand between the flange and my breast. It was almost as if he were saying, "You're stealing my milk. Give it back now!"

And here's the really ironic part: I'd freeze that stash of 'liquid gold' to no avail. He didn't like the thawed-out milk! Time and again I'd try to get him to drink his milk from a bottle, only with minimal success. We didn't supplement (as my oldest ended up having a dairy allergy and we just weren't sure if Elijah would have the same issue). We just kept trying. Somehow it all worked out and now he enjoys almond milk just like his other brothers—he even asks for seconds!

Heather's Story: Feeders

Anecdote

Just a few days after my daughter Tiernan was born, I took my older daughter Ryan (3½) out for ice cream and a little mommy/daughter time, just the two of us. We went to Dairy Queen, had our ice cream, and then I let her romp in the play place for awhile. After about an hour I told her we needed to get home because mommy needed to feed baby sister.

She stopped and looked at me, totally serious-like, pointed her finger at me with authority and said, "Because you've got the feeders, right?"

I said yes, and so we packed up and left. On the way home, she continued, "Does Daddy have feeders?"

"No," I replied.

"I've got feeders," she said. "But mine are too small. Only mommies have big feeders."

Nobody Said it Would be Easy (Thankfully)

I really appreciated the honest moms who told me, "It isn't always easy!" I've had two little girls and two completely different experiences. One took to breastfeeding immediately and we sailed through months with no problems. The other was harder; but knowing that just because it was hard didn't mean it wasn't going to work really helped me stick with it—and every day, every week it got easier! So just because it isn't easy at first or just because it might be difficult doesn't mean every experience is going to be the same. Stick with it if you can.

Before my first daughter was born, I knew I wanted to breastfeed but was really afraid that it wouldn't feel natural to me—that it would feel weird or that I was too modest to do it. But my own mother really reassured me, telling me again and again that God designed women (and not just humans, but all mammals) to nurse their young. She said that once my baby and I were able to establish breastfeeding, nothing would feel more special or natural. She was right. I found nothing more comforting or calming than snuggling my baby against me, our warm bodies touching, and feeding her. I gave her what she needs from me and created that special bond at the same time.

Tips

One of the best tips I have to give is that if you need to pump a bottle, do it at the same time you are nursing. I get a good latch with my baby and let her start eating on one breast, then I hook up the pump on the other breast and turn it on. I get almost twice the milk for my bottle this way!

Once you are home from the hospital, the first few days should be all about connecting. When you have to nurse, do your best to go somewhere you can be alone with your baby; get comfortable and quiet; and bond. Breastfeeding can be difficult and painful those first few days and the more calm you are the better and EASIER it will be for you and baby to make it work.

Jen's Story: Note to Self

My husband and I were at the hospital waiting on some final paperwork before being discharged. We decided it would be a perfect time to try and pump because the lactation specialist told us that pumping would keep the breasts stimulated for milk production.

As I pumped, Nathan and I marveled at the various dials and buttons. I asked him what he thought the dial was for, and after replying that he didn't know, I told him to twist it. It seemed like a good idea at the time.

The next thing I know, my breasts were being sucked into the tubing like a vacuum! I jumped up off the bed screaming, "Turn it off! Turn it off!" Nathan started pushing buttons and twisting dials in a panic. I finally broke the seal from my breasts and pulled them off. We laughed so hard we had tears in our eyes!

Note to self: always read the instructions first!

Stories of Wisdom

A wise attitude, belief, or course of action.

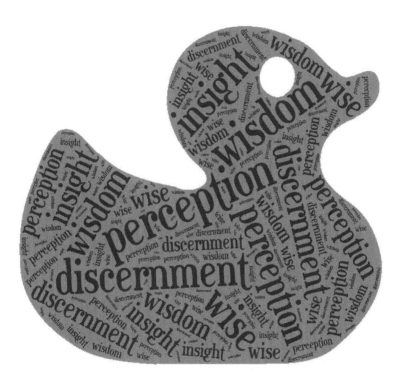

Holly's Story:
The Best Laid Plans

When I was pregnant with my first child I went to a breastfeeding class, but admittedly, I only half listened. I was sure that I would be able to nurse my child without a problem because women had been doing it for centuries. On top of that, my boobs had quadrupled in size, so I felt I was bound to be able to produce plenty of milk. All I really needed to do was have my baby, use my purple tube of lanolin (a kernel of wisdom I did pick up from breastfeeding class), possibly use the football hold (the other thing I learned), and lovingly offer my breast to my baby and that would be that. I would join the ranks of all of the women who chose to nurse their babies. Piece of cake.

That thought changed after an exhausting three-day attempt at a traditional delivery with lots of futile pushing, throwing up, and a fever. I ended up with an emergency C-section. Not long after, I was handed my infant daughter and was told it was time to feed her. I remember feeling like I had been hit by a train from the birthing experience; fumbling around with my breasts; juggling an increasingly frustrated, crying baby; and doing what I could to get things to connect. I couldn't get it to work. By this time, I was sweating, my husband was looking panicky, the baby's cries had gone up several decibels, and my boobs were too slobbery and slippery from our many failed attempts at nursing to secure a good latch even if I could have figured it out. Fortunately, the lactation consultant was nearby and came in to rescue my poor baby and me. That was when I learned that I had flat nipples. What? "Of course your baby can't latch on, honey, you have flat nipples," the lactation consultant informed me over the sound of my wailing baby. With a lot of pinching, mostly on the part of the consultant because at that point I had given up control of my boobs to the expert, she managed to get my baby to latch on. Hallelujah! The room was quiet again. I could catch my breath and let my blood pressure get back to normal. I think my husband would have kissed the woman if he had had the chance. We were so grateful to be able to finally feed our baby.

Unbeknownst to me, nipples are not one size fits all. Following my initial ordeal, the lactation consultant was able to show me how to pinch and squeeze my breast/nipple in order for it to be less flat and therefore fit into my baby's mouth better. After about a week of breastfeeding, my nipples took on a whole new shape and I didn't have to worry about it anymore. Thankfully I was able to breastfeed my baby without too much trouble once the whole flat nipple thing was resolved. But it certainly wasn't quite the piece of cake I was expecting.

I am now the mother of four and have nursed each of my girls for around a year and am currently nursing my last little guy who is 15 months old. Below I have compiled some of the things I've learned about breastfeeding. Hopefully they will help you succeed at nursing your own baby, or at the very least, help you feel not so alone in your own flat nipple experience.

Advice

- ***Nursing bras***. Get fitted for some good nursing bras when you are within a month or two of your due date. You won't be able to imagine your breasts getting any larger than they already have, but don't be fooled, you will increase in size another two-fold when your milk comes in. In my case, I started out as a full C cup before pregnancy and gradually became a very full D cup towards the end of my last trimester. When I went shopping for bras, I bought three that were D cups and one double E cup nursing bra that the sales woman talked me into. I kept my receipt for the BIG bra because I doubted I would ever get that BIG. When my milk actually came in, I could barely squeeze into my BIG bra. I only needed it for about three weeks and then my breasts regulated themselves according to my baby's needs, but I was really glad to have it for that time.

  I found front snap nursing bras to be easier to maneuver when nursing in public. They also kept my nursing pad more in place, so it was less likely to flip out onto the sidewalk when I was trying to be discrete about breastfeeding in places with lots of people. If it does happen to flip out, just kick the pad under your seat and pick it up when you are done feeding your baby. I speak from experience on this one. It's also a good idea to keep a spare pad in your baby bag, just in case you have leaky boobs like mine and your pad goes flying out unexpectedly. Speaking of flying nursing pads, Johnsons® makes a great disposable pad that has a little sticky part that secures it to the inside of your bra. These pads are super leak proof, too.

- **Lanolin.** Lanolin is <u>very</u> important in keeping your nipples from becoming overly sore. I always took a tube with me to the hospital and when I came home I had two tubes: one upstairs and one downstairs. You will be sore regardless of using lanolin, but it helps keep your nipples from feeling terribly raw. A little bit on the very tips of your nipples is perfect. Use it frequently, before and after breastfeeding. I also put it on before I got into the shower for the first few weeks I started nursing. Make sure you don't go overboard with using it, though. With my second born, I was feeling so sore one evening that I slathered it all over my nipples and areolas wondering if I shouldn't just rub it all over my body to see if it would help ease my pain. In the end, I had created a waxy, slippery situation that prevented my baby from getting latched on at all when she was hungry! I ended up in the bathroom with a washcloth, feverishly trying to wipe off the lanolin while my baby screamed in the next room. Lesson learned.

- **Energizer Bunny.** Try to keep it down to only nursing for 20-30 minutes on each side when you start out breastfeeding. Your baby will want to suck forever, but your nipples will have a hard time forgiving you if you let that happen. I remember sitting up practically all night at the hospital one night with my first born letting her stay latched onto my breasts for as long as she wanted. I was going to feed her really well and be the best mom ever. Fortunately, I shared my joy about this feat with the lactation consultant the next day and she was quick to correct my mistake. When my pain meds wore off, I knew exactly what she was talking about.

- ***Engorged!*** Using a breast pump is a great way to alleviate how swollen your breasts get once your milk comes in. If your breasts get so full that they are tight, which tends to happen in the first week, your baby will have a hard time latching on. If I didn't have a chance to pump out a little bit before I needed to nurse, I used a pacifier for a minute to placate the baby, letdown my milk, let it flow into a burp cloth for a few seconds to get my breasts back to a supple point, and then had the baby latch on.

- ***Just Don't Burst a Capillary.*** A side note about pumping in the early weeks: your breasts can be sensitive to pumping and you can inadvertently burst a capillary along your milk ducts—which then causes blood to mix in with your milk. You may not know this is happening, and it's not harmful to the baby if it does. It will, however, freak you out to see blood in your 5 day old baby's spit up and cause you to rush off to the ER without the ability to speak through your uncontrollable tears. Yes, this happened to me and it was a nightmare that turned out to be not such a big deal after all. Apparently it's not so unusual—even though it had never happened to me or anyone I knew of before. Now you know.

- ***Tired!*** Don't be surprised if you feel really sleepy—like someone knocked you over the head with a frying pan sleepy—when you are breastfeeding for the first week or so. I remember being completely alert and conversation worthy until about five minutes after I began nursing my baby and then it was everything I could do to keep my eyes open. As your baby sucks, he/she stimulates your pituitary gland which then releases the hormone Oxytocin which in turn can make you feel calm, relaxed, and *very* sleepy. Your body eventually gets used to this and your husband won't have to worry about being a bore.

- *Positioning is Key*. Sit up as straight as you can when you are nursing. Put a pillow behind your back to give you support and straighten out your posture. This helps put your body into alignment so that juggling your baby is a little easier as you get him/her latched on. It also helped me to keep my baby in a comfortable position and it allowed me to better monitor the way he/she was latched on. For example, two out of four of my babies liked to wheedle their way to the very tip of my nipple instead of keeping the whole mouthful.

Make sure you have your baby in a "belly to belly" position when you nurse. I remember feeding my first newborn one morning and noticing that her poor little neck was completely cranked to the side because her body was flat on my lap. Once I flipped her floppy body close to mine, belly to belly, she was able to snuggle in better and nursed more comfortably. This was a light bulb moment for me as a first time mom. Using a nursing pillow or fluffy blanket on your lap is also helpful to get a good nursing position.

- **Baby Bird Phenomenon**. Move your baby to your breast, not your breast to your baby. My husband and I refer to this as the "baby bird" phenomenon. Here's how it goes: I would cradle my baby, tickle his/her mouth with my nipple to get him/her to open really wide (think baby robin) to get a big mouthful of nipple (or worm in a bird's case) and then pull my baby up and into a latch on my breast. The other way around can lead to sore nipples because of the position you put yourself in as the baby latches on.

- **Latch**. Make sure your baby <u>does not</u> wheedle his/her way down to the nub of your nipple. You will be sore afterwards. A full mouthful of nipple is the best way to go. If you have a wheedling baby, unlatch and re-latch every time it happens. Sometimes I had to interrupt nursing my baby several times in order to get back to a good latch. The baby will eventually get used to the idea and you will both be better for it.

- **Parched**. Have a large glass of water within reach of wherever you are planning to breastfeed your baby, especially at night. You will be unbelievably parched as you nurse, and having water at hand is such a relief. For the first few months, I always put a giant water bottle on the nightstand next to the rocking chair in the nursery before I went to bed so it was ready when I needed it during the middle of the night feedings. Keeping well hydrated is also a key to keeping your milk supply steady.

- ***Nothing but Air.*** Understand that having sore nipples is normal and it happens with each and every child you breastfeed. I had hoped that when I had my second child that my nipples would have been toughened up by my first baby, but no such luck. They weren't flat anymore, though. Using lanolin helps and calling your hospital's lactation consultant for advice after you have gone home and you're sad about being sore is also a good idea. The other thing that is crucial to helping sore nipples recover is to make sure they get lots of air time. I was given some plastic, turtle shell-looking cups to slip into my bra by my lactation consultant when I was in the hospital with my fourth child. They initially were meant to help women who had inverted nipples—another wonder—but also could be used to allow air to circulate around the nipple even with a bra and shirt on. Genius! They made my breasts appear to be even more ridiculous than they already were, but they helped cut down on the soreness I had developed in a big way. The other thing I did that helped was to lift my shirt up when I was sleeping at night so that my breasts could air out. Forget sleeping on your side or stomach when you have two gigantic cantaloupes on your chest in the first place, so just let those babies out in the open for the few minutes/hours you get to put your head on your pillow. It will make a difference, I promise.

- ***Good News!*** You will not be sore forever. It will become natural and pain free in about 3-4 weeks from the day you start breastfeeding. It's hard to imagine this day when you are curling your toes from the pain of each latch, but it will come. Don't give up! I take full credit in how smart my children are and for the very few ear infections they have had to suffer all because I breastfed them. Yep, I did it.

- **Not Tonight.** Don't worry when your libido is lost and nowhere to be found. It will come back when you are down to only a few feedings or completely finished breastfeeding. Think of it as Mother Nature's birth control. Cut out the desire part and the mother stays focused on her baby's survival. I didn't know what was up with me when I had my first child, and I wish someone would have mentioned this. It's also helpful information for your husband, so he doesn't have his feelings hurt if you turn down his passes. And remember, you can still get pregnant when you're breastfeeding, so don't let it fool you.

- **Mastitis.** Mastitis is nothing to sneeze at. I've had it three times. Know the symptoms (unusual pain nursing, low grade fever, red streaks on your breast, fever in the breast) and if you even think you have it, call your doctor. Wake them up at night if you have to and find an all-night pharmacy to get your antibiotics if necessary. It's a big deal to get it treated right away. Keep on nursing through it, too. It helps.

- **Food.** Your diet makes a difference with your breast milk. I found that my babies were especially gassy and hard to soothe when I had eaten anything green (salad, broccoli, green beans, etc.), spicy foods (pepperoni pizza,

Mexican), and/or dairy products (ice cream, milk, cheese). If I cut these types of foods out of my diet for the first three months of breastfeeding, my baby had fewer painful gas episodes. Somewhere around 4 months, I was able to introduce these foods back into my diet without much trouble caused to the baby. Mylicon® Infant Gas Drops are extremely helpful when your baby has gas issues and you can't just pop the bubbles with a few extra pats on the back.

Breastfeeding can be hard and complicated for sure. It is not the piece of cake I originally thought it would be. But it is one of my absolute favorite parts of being a mother. I love the closeness, the snuggle-up time with my baby, and the milky grins. I love how it makes me stop what I'm doing so I can do nothing but pay attention to my baby. Rocking my baby as he quietly nurses and then so contentedly falls asleep in my arms is priceless. It's also very empowering to be able to instantly calm your baby with your body when he is in distress. Not to mention how convenient it is to have something to nourish your baby with wherever you go—for free. I don't think I'll ever be able to give away my creaky old glider because of the memories I have had in it with each of my children. Breastfeeding is a wonderful experience you will be happy you chose to do...once you get the hang of it.

Wendy's Story: Mother Nature Knows Best

My husband and I went through the nursing classes prior to our first child's birth. As a very modest and private person, I needed as much support as I could get. I was very nervous about nursing, and it was helpful having my husband in the classes so he could support me through the emotions and techniques associated with breastfeeding.

Emma was born on Easter Sunday with jaundice. Therefore she was very reluctant to eat and much more willing to sleep. My first attempts at nursing required some adjustments as I tried to find a position that was comfortable for me and still allowed her to latch on. When the lactation consultant visited, she kept insisting that I push more of my breast into Emma's mouth. When you're a 34M (marble) there is not much extra to work with, and it was very frustrating for me! Eventually we figured it out, and Emma would latch on and suckle. She would soon nod off to sleep, and in my exhausted state I would soon follow. This was the fairy tale as I thought it would play out.

While at the hospital, they would bring Emma to me about every three hours to nurse. We had to tickle her feet, undress her, and change her diaper just to try and keep her awake. They became very concerned because Emma was losing weight rather than gaining. I soon learned there was a product (called a Supplemental Nursing System®) that supplements your child while nursing so your baby will gain weight, and decided I would give it a try. I looked like I was getting ready to blast off—with a small tube that was attached to liquid formula that I had to put next to my breast while nursing. The tube also did not help in finding comfortable nursing positions. We still had to work at keeping Emma awake while nursing. So much for the fairy tale. In addition, the lactation consultant and nurses informed me I had to wake her up in the middle of the night for feedings. These nightly wake ups did not sit well with Emma; and she would let us know by staying awake for *hours* after the feeding.

We stayed an extra day but were sent home with instructions to continue the feeding routine—even through the night—and to keep her in the sunlight as much as possible to alleviate the jaundice.

In the 48 hours that followed, I became increasingly desperate for Emma to eat a full meal. I did not feel like I was doing it right because she would only eat for a minute or two and would now often fuss during the feedings—especially the night feedings. I tried every hold, I tried both breasts, I called the doctor, and I called the lactation consultant. The experts just told me to stick to the schedule and keep working at it. Now I was engorged, sleep deprived, and getting very irritable!

It all ended one afternoon when my husband walked in from feeding our horses to hear my mom and I trying to console a fussy Emma. I could not keep her awake to eat and she was not latching on at all. My mother informed me to ignore the expert advice and quit waking Emma up at night. She was of the camp that said you never wake a sleeping baby. Then, much to my mother's horror, my husband opened the blinds to the large picture window in our living room and pointed to the pasture where several cows were grazing while their calves slept. He pointed out the window and said, "You see those calves over there? They sleep when they're tired, they poop when they need to, and they eat when they are hungry." He told me to put Emma down and let her sleep. She immediately went to sleep and I again worked on perfecting my breast-pumping techniques. When she woke up, she was quite hungry and I was relieved when she latched on perfectly! That night at bedtime we did not wake her up for a feeding. My husband and I awoke at five the next morning frightened. We had all slept through the night...including Emma! We rushed to her room and saw a peaceful little Easter present resting.

From that point forward, Emma only ate once a night and quickly moved to meals during the day only. Now I understand what Mother Nature already knew: the experts can assist, but you have to do what works for you and your baby.

Emma is now always hungry, sleeps through the night, and is always up first in the morning.

Lynn's Story: The Non-Milk Diary

I won't ever forget the day that changed my life. Many women may assume my answer would be the day I gave birth to my first child. Although that day was huge in the history of days, the day I'm remembering is the day that some kind soul at a lactation support meeting came up to me and suggested my daughter may have a food allergy or sensitivity. I was the mom in the back of the room with a screaming three-week old baby girl. She had been screaming since two days after she was born. The pediatrician told me it was "colic" and that she would outgrow it by three months old.

The woman who helped me that day wasn't a lactation consultant. She was just a mom, like you and like me, who had gone through a screaming baby and figured out what was wrong and lived to tell about it. She explained the symptoms of a cow's milk protein intolerance and helped me find some literature that explained how to take milk protein out of my diet for a 2-week food trial to see if that was what was bothering my baby. I took home the list of foods and food additives I could no longer eat and set forth trying to make a meal plan for the next week. I was amazed at how immediately we saw results. My baby still cried occasionally, but she was much different than the screaming-every-waking-moment baby that we brought home from the hospital. When I told my pediatrician what I was doing, she suggested that we try a hypo-allergenic formula instead. That didn't make any sense to me. It was well worth the personal sacrifice on my part to not eat or drink milk protein if my baby would be happier and not in pain. I didn't want the cost or trouble of formula, and who knew what was in that hypo-allergenic stuff anyway?

My daughter is now 8 and has no food allergies or sensitivities thanks to the wisdom of another mom—coupled with advice from wonderful lactation consultants.

When our second child was born, we knew right away that he had a sensitive tummy, too. I immediately gave up milk protein again, with mixed results. I went to see my lactation consultant and she told me about a new (at the time) phenomenon they were seeing in babies. It was called M.S.P.I., or milk-soy protein intolerance. I had been consuming a lot of soy (milk, tofu) as a substitute for milk, and it was making my baby sick. His diapers tested positive for blood in the bowel movements. I gave up eating soy protein, and again, the results were nearly miraculous. The blood was gone from his diaper, and he was a much happier baby. In fact, he was the happiest baby I've had—sleeping well at night and contented.

It was an easy decision to give up milk and soy when our third child was born, just as a precaution. My plan was to slowly introduce them into my diet as she got a little bigger, but that day took a while to come. Soon after birth, my midwife contacted me about being a private milk donor for an adopted baby with a serious allergy to milk protein. I went through a couple simple health tests, primed my pump, and began to pump for my donor baby. I've always had oversupply, so it was easy! Many weeks I was pumping 100 ounces in addition to exclusively feeding my plump nursling. And the mama, oh, was she happy to get this donor milk to feed her baby! I benefited, too, because I didn't ever suffer from engorgement. Both babies thrived and we donated milk for almost ten months.

Many thanks to my early lactation consultants at Milkworks in Lincoln, Nebraska. Not only did they help me fix two "colicky" babies, they taught me how to wear my babies and about attachment parenting. I "pay it forward" to new mommies every chance I get.

I am now happily expecting baby #5 and can't wait to nurse again!

Catherine's Story: One of These Kids is Not Like the Other

By the time I was ready to deliver my third child, I thought that I had breastfeeding all figured out. I had breastfed my first two daughters and had come through on the other side with growing babies and breasts intact. Sure, there was plenty of difficulty and drama, but in general, it was a positive experience. When my third daughter arrived, she latched on like a professional. The nurses would pop in and comment on how great she was doing. The lactation consultant came by and confirmed this. She praised me and my baby on our success. I felt so blessed to have this amazing and healthy little girl who made our family complete. I felt doubly blessed that the breastfeeding just seemed to be so effortless and natural. But it didn't stay that way for long.

In the first few weeks after her birth, my baby and I developed a bit of a latching problem. My nipples were red, sore, and uncomfortable; the pain was toe curling at times. I stuck it out for several days and tried to convince myself that it would get better and my baby and I would find our rhythm again with each other any minute. But we didn't. She seemed happy, but I was miserable. Let me rephrase that: my breasts were miserable. I swallowed a big gulp of pride and set up an appointment with one of the lactation consultants at the hospital.

After I showed the consultant how I would normally nurse my baby, she made a few slight adjustments to our positioning. Within moments, I felt comfortable and the nursing felt right again. It amazed me how little it took to make such a huge difference.

I had a conversation with her about how stupid I felt that I had to be there in the first place. I shared with her that I had two other children and that by now, I should really have this thing down. I felt sad and insecure that I hadn't had nursing mastered already. I guess I felt like a bit of a failure. The confident woman and mom I envisioned myself to be was having a hard time admitting that she needed help.

So to all you moms who are struggling with nursing, take it easy on yourself. Ask for help (I recommend these lactation consultants—they are such a great resource!). Babies are unique individuals and they all have their own little preferences from the day they are born. Sometimes it just takes a little bit of tweaking to get it right, even if you have done it a couple times before.

Mary Ellen's Story: Top Ten Tips for Long-term Success

1. A nursing stool in the hospital room is helpful! With my first I tried to make do with a wastebasket on its side. Not good.

2. Those Lily Padz® nursing pads work pretty well. I liked not having something to throw away all the time.

3. Cracked and bleeding nipples do HURT. I never had time to do all those things they tell you to do (like showers and cabbage leaves or tea). My sister's comment to "slather on the lanolin" was the most helpful. (She also told me she said the rosary while nursing to help her through it.)

4. Learning the side-lying position made a HUGE difference for me, allowing me to sleep while nursing.

5. You CAN nurse a child with teeth. They can learn not to bite. They're just playing when they do it (at least at first—when they are three, they know darn well what they're doing).

6. I've known people to use breast milk as medicine, dripping it on pink-eye or rashes.

7. It would be good to teach your child a slightly disguised way to ask to nurse. I didn't do this soon enough. Son #1 didn't talk when I nursed him, and son #2 started talking before I got the code ready. I think the best thing is to call it milk, so you can just ask, "Do you want some milk?" and no one listening knows what you really mean.

8. La Leche League is an excellent resource. The Womanly Art of Breastfeeding is a great book.

9. I have nursed in so many places and situations I can hardly think of anywhere I haven't. I nursed a child in a car seat while we were both strapped in. I even switched sides! I nursed in church (though I didn't like that too much by the time they were good walkers). I nursed in front of high school students when I was a teacher (just once). I've nursed on the toilet. I've nursed in the library. I nursed on the train at the zoo. I've nursed on airplanes. And I never had anyone complain to me about it in person. Usually people would rather see a contented child than a screaming one, so if nursing is what was needed, that's what I did.

10. Nursing has so many benefits I don't know why more moms don't try it. Yes, I had some challenges (and pain), but the positives are so much greater! Healthy kids getting exactly what they need, no expensive formula, no period for months, quick weight loss (in my case, at least), no need to carry much with you when out with baby (or need to find a good water supply or heating device), and lowered risk of cancer for mom. I'm sure you can add many more to this list.

Lanee's Story: Working Mama

The Beginning

Although I breastfed my babies some, I mostly pumped. I didn't come to this decision just because I planned to go back to work. You see, Parker was really gassy and would only breastfeed about 5 minutes at a time and then would play with my nipple for the remaining 10 to 20 minutes. He would then proceed to spit up a lot of milk and want to eat again in 45 minutes! Every hour was too much to handle, so eating from a bottle seemed to work best for us—even when I was at home. I also say the best bottles in the world are the wide mouth Dr. Brown Natural Flow® bottles (make sure you buy wide mouth). They have a lot of parts, but it is worth the hassle.

My advice would be to start saving milk early after week 2. I waited to store milk until the recommended 4 weeks, but was having difficulty making enough milk to feed Parker *and* store some for when I went back to work. If you try to increase your milk supply earlier than later, you may avoid supplementing with formula during the growth spurts.

Growth Spurt Warnings

Hopefully you gals can breastfeed successfully through the growth spurts. My friend Melissa suggests having your husband change baby's diaper and bring him to you to nurse at night. Then you can get more rest between feedings—especially the first 6 weeks.

Parker slept a lot the first two weeks, but the two growth spurts during that timeframe were hard to work through. It was hard to keep up with the every 2-3 hour round-the-clock feedings from weeks 2 ½ through 3 ½ (yielding about 2-3 ounces). And week 5 to week 7 was another hard time (yielding 4½-5½ ounces). The Nursing Mother's Companion book tells you how much to bottle breastfeed your baby and provides a helpful chart to figure out how many ounces your baby needs. That was super helpful to me to ensure baby was getting enough.

Frozen Gold

Here's an alternative to buying specialty nursing bags that my friend Kerri told me about. Store 2-4 ounces of milk in a pint-size freezer bag (warning: over 4 ounces will leak!) Next, you can put five of the pint-size freezer bags in 1 gallon-size freezer bag before placing milk in a deepfreeze. Lay the bags flat in the freezer. The breast milk stays good for 3 months in a refrigerator freezer and for up to one year in a deepfreeze. Pump every 3-4 hours to maintain milk; to increase milk supply, try pumping every 2-3 hours. Pumping and cleaning bottles takes a lot of time, but going back to work will require a lot of stored milk!

Breastfeeding Position

The traditional breastfeeding positions caused Parker to choke and vomit. The books I read only had traditional breastfeeding positions. I was about to give up on breastfeeding and only pump when I finally found a new breastfeeding position. If you want to see this position in action, visit the website http://www.kellymom.com/bf/supply/fast-letdown.html. It sure helped me!

Mona's Story: Sometimes Less is More

Let me preface by saying I may be the most flat-chested woman on Earth. So I always figured that if I had a baby, my baby would probably starve. Boy was I wrong!

My little girl was placed in the NICU due to respiratory distress soon after she was born. My milk had not come in yet, but the nurses stressed pumping whenever possible to build up my milk supply. (In hindsight, I'm thinking that was a big cause of my OVERPRODUCTION.) By the end of the first week of birth, I could produce six ounces from one breast in five minutes!!!!!! Yes, you read that correctly…that's twelve ounces at one pumping! I could have single-handedly fed a small infant army.

Now I'm sure some think this would be awesome, but let me assure you that it is anything but. Going from barely an A cup to DD cups of insane pain and milk squirting in all directions at the mere cry of a baby across town is NOT fun. This began a vicious cycle of awful pain, blocked milk ducts, and eventual mastitis. To make matters worse, since my baby couldn't handle all the milk, she would only latch on if I had pumped a few minutes prior to feeding—making me produce even more milk. UGH!!! And after each feeding, my baby would subsequently vomit most of her meal back up on my shoulder. I spent many a feeding crying and then cleaning up vomit.

It wasn't until around three months later (and a LOT of full breast pads) when a lactation consultant suggest that I stop pumping all together and put red cabbage leaves in my bra that I began to tolerate breastfeeding. My production did slow down, but I still had plenty of milk. After my first child turned one, I threw out four gallons of frozen breast milk from my deepfreeze.

Please don't take this as a sob story to knock breastfeeding; instead, use it as a learning tool. It IS possible for a flat-chested woman to [over]produce breast milk. And it is possible to manage production with a little help from a consultant. I breastfed my first baby until she was eight months old and my second till he was six months old. All the pain didn't deter me because I knew it was the healthiest choice for my situation. But I won't say it was easy.

Sherri's Story: Goal-Oriented People Find Ways

Breastfeeding is the ONE thing you and only you can give your baby. It may not have been the easiest thing I've ever done, but it was definitely the most selfless thing.

Advice

- The main thing is not to let the nurses at the hospital scare you. They do this day in and day out and will just grab that baby and stick her on your boob...they can be very abrupt. They do care for your baby; they just know she's not going to break.

- Stick to your plans. Do not let a family member or nurse influence you. Many moms today are the first generation to breastfeed. Grandmothers, aunts, sisters, and sisters-in-law sometimes just don't understand why you are doing it. Besides the big boobs, it is still one of the neatest, coolest things I have ever done for my child. Plus, I really do think she is smart because of it and she has never had an ear infection.

- Set goals for yourself. First just get through the hospital stay. Then set a goal for one week at home. Then one month...then each month after. Soon you will be to six months and your body will be a machine.

- Go out for a drink with your husband a few times. It is OK to pump and dump.

- Your plans may not work exactly how you intended—you might have the child that just doesn't get the latching or sucking thing. Things will get better—just give it time.

Grab this Gear!

- Breast pumps are something I knew nothing about. You can buy a used machine on eBay or Craig's List and save yourself hundreds of dollars, or borrow from a friend. (Just make sure to give that friend a gift card at the end—they saved you a lot of money!) All you need to buy new are the horn things and tubes. The breast milk never goes through the actual machine.

- Get a Boppy® pillow! This is the best arm-saving device for breastfeeding moms.

- I was a working mom and still to this day think nursing shirts are the best invention ever! I could feed without even pulling a blanket out. There would be people coming up to my baby that had no clue I was breastfeeding. THESE SHIRTS ROCK! They made life SOOOOO much easier! Trust me.

Kerri's Story: Breastfeeding is Not for Sissies

There were a couple of things that prepared me to breastfeed:

- A very supportive friend who breastfed before me.

- Ambition and perseverance for achieving the goals I set.

Every new mother needs a friend to call—someone's shoulder to cry on or ask for advice or to tell "I want to give up!" when you really don't. Without that friend, it's so easy to just quit. Let's face it: guys can't possibly understand what it's like to have a baby stuck to your boob for what seems like 24/7, the pain of a fissure splitting your nipple in half, engorgement, clogged ducts, or the soreness from a newborn learning to suckle. Nor do most of our mothers, from what I've gathered. Most of my friends were bottle fed as infants. Our mothers knew all the tricks to dry the milk up but no clue how to keep the wells open. At least for me, the success of my breastfeeding was dependent upon the support of my friend, Sherri (see her story on page 169). When I said I couldn't do it, she said I could and I should. When I was in pain, she listened to me cry. When I was exhausted, she let me complain. When my production decreased, she researched methods to increase my supply. As much as my husband tried to support me, his idea of *supporting* me was telling me to quit—which was the last thing I wanted to hear. I wanted to hear, "You can do it. I love you. You are so amazing. Our son is so lucky to have a mom like you." Not so much.

Setting Short-term Goals

When I was nursing, the AAP recommended nursing for at least the first year. But when in the midst of the fatigue, pain, frustration—a year seems like eternity! I set shorter goals—the first six weeks (and actually, everything gets a lot easier after that), then it was until I went back to work. Once returning to work, it was four months (which is a third of a year!), then six months (halfway there...woo hoo!). After that, I took it day by day. Unfortunately, with my son, I began to dry up and working ten hour days did not help. I was blessed enough to have nursed him for nine months. And with my frozen supply, my son was fed a combination of formula/breast milk for just under a year.

Every Baby Can be Different

I read every book about babies with my son, and it seems the theme was schedule, schedule, schedule! So like the books suggested, I tried to get my boobs and my baby on the same schedule. After a lot of frustration, the schedule approach failed for many reasons. First, I was timid, shy, modest, and almost embarrassed to nurse in public or even in another room at family homes. So I would bring bottles of milk with me if we had errands to run or family functions and then pump or feed when I got home. When I went back to work, I worked three 10-hour days. I attempted to get my son and boobs on my "work" pump schedule and bottle feed at the same time on my days off. But the planning and trying to stick to an unrealistic and difficult schedule was very stressful! Maybe that's why my wells dried up with my son.

So when my daughter was born, I threw the whole schedule and expert's knowledge out the window! No longer was I worried about every two-hour feedings, alternating boobs, or letting a four-week-old helpless Godly creature cry it out because she would be spoiled otherwise! Heck no! I let the boobies hang out and let freedom ring! Women's lib 2006! Well, not so much, but I did let go of the embarrassment of breastfeeding. I embraced the natural God-given gift only a woman could provide. For the first six months of my baby girl's life, she needed nothing but her mommy's milk (and love, of course) to survive. I never exposed myself (at least not intentionally, but I'm sure some innocent bystanders got an eyeful). I kept my shawl with me and nursed whenever and wherever baby girl demanded. Bye bye schedule! No more bottles, no more stress, no more worrying where I would be when letdown occurred. Besides, with a very active toddler in hand, I would have had a nervous breakdown stuck in the home with an infant stuck to my boobs!

I exuded more confidence and felt proud. Baby girl did not eat anything but mommy's milk for the first six months of her life. How awesome is that?!?!? I nursed her in the middle of a mall at Christmas time, on a train at the zoo, while shopping at

Target, bagging groceries at Shop 'n Save, at the playground, at the pool...you name it.

Circumstances do change between each child, but letting go of the structure enhanced my nursing experience with my second child. It no longer seemed like a job. It felt more natural and definitely more enjoyable. Maybe it's because I had prior experience or maybe it's because my outlook on nursing changed. Nursing was no longer just about setting and reaching a goal...nursing was a once in a lifetime bonding experience with my baby. And in my opinion, there isn't anything in this world that could ever compare.

Just Some Thoughts

- It's ok to cry over spilled milk. Most likely you will, and people will look at you like you are crazy. Breast milk is like gold and you worked hard for every ounce you pump...and only you can produce the specialized formula for your baby. I once had a meltdown when I spilled a 2 oz bottle!

- I calculated that I spent approximately eight hours per day during the first 6-8 weeks of my son's life with nursing and everything associated with pumping. Nurse, pump, package milk in bags to freeze, clean bottles and shields, dry, boil tea bags (awesome remedy for sore nipples!), then repeat 6-7 times per day.

- My children each preferred a different breast. My son preferred the right while my daughter preferred the left.

For three years, my right breast sagged about two inches lower than my left. After baby girl, both breasts sagged evenly and are now proportionate to each other once again (thank goodness for Victoria's Secret!).

- I ruined 400 thread count sheets from leaking boobs in the middle of the night. I had to sleep with towels under my boobs due to the constant outflow of milk. My breasts were so full and hard I would have to pump first before my son nursed just so he could latch on. On the contrary, I rarely felt letdown with my daughter. I never felt my milk "come in" for the first time or experienced the engorgement of milk. Yet, I produced more milk with her.

- My toddler once brought a bottle of expressed breast milk from the refrigerator when my four-week old baby was crying and said, "Here Mommy. You need to put this in your booby. My baby sister is crying."

- A nurse in the hospital gave me the tip of using regular freezer bags instead of the breast milk bags for storage. 1. It's cheaper. 2. They store more easily because they lay flat in the freezer, and allow more room. I froze 2-4 ounces in a sandwich size bag and then double-bagged 5-6 sandwich bags in one gallon freezer bag. Each individual bag thaws quickly under warm water. Snip the corner of the bag with scissors to easily empty contents into a bottle!

I was fortunate enough to have my grandparents watch both of my babies when I worked. I never had to worry about diaper bags, change of clothes, bottles, etc. because I brought a supply of everything to keep over there. They also had a deep freeze which became my personal breast milk storage facility! I never had to worry about making sure I had enough milk pumped for the day. My grandparents kept the frozen supply and would thaw the milk as they needed. Once my freezer would fill up, I would pack a cooler of frozen milk and stock up my grandparent's freezer. I had a continual and consistent supply of milk with my baby girl and little of the reserves were needed. I would have loved to have donated my precious commodity to a milk bank but was unable to. It took my grandpa almost a whole day to drain all of my "liquid gold" – with many mixed emotions from me: sadness to see it all go to waste…embarrassment with my grandpa handling all of my milk!

Beth's Story: Last But Not Least

Work and my First Two Babies

When I had my first two kids, I worked full time. My goal was to nurse them for a year each while pumping at work. I had no idea how hard pumping was going to be. I didn't build up a supply before I went back to work and struggled to pump enough during the day to provide for the next. I made the decision with each of them to supplement with formula. I still pumped, but once the breast milk was gone, the daycare workers used formula. This was a hard decision to make initially but it was the best one given the circumstances. I stopped stressing over the amount of milk I was able to pump and just reminded myself that even a little was better than none.

Last but not Least

When I had my third child, I just assumed nursing her would be as easy as it was with my first two. When she was born, I wanted to start nursing her right away, but somehow having a C-section and my tubes tied got in the way. Those procedures earned me a double dose of morphine which made me very, very sick. I reluctantly agreed to let her have formula that first night. The next day we tried nursing again, and she nursed like a champ! For about five minutes. She then fell fast asleep and wouldn't wake up. I was so tired myself that I just let her sleep. About 1 ½ hours later, she was hungry again and nursed on the other side. For a whopping 5 minutes.

So the pattern began: this girl was definitely a snacker, and I was getting increasingly frustrated. At about 3 weeks old, she started crying from about 5:00 PM-10:00 PM straight. Nothing would calm her: she would neither eat nor sleep. During this time I was at my wit's end. I was still trying to nurse her, but we would both get so upset. I was in tears. I finally realized that I couldn't nurse her when I was so upset; I would have to walk away. I would put her in her swing or give her to daddy and just leave the house for a few minutes. Once I was able to get some fresh air and take a deep breath, I was able to relax and try to nurse her again.

I also learned the value of having her on a schedule. I was completely opposed to that idea with my first two but realized this child was different! I started forcing her to nurse a full 10 minutes on each side at each feeding (which I determined—not her). I did whatever it took to keep her awake. I would strip her down to her diaper, rub cool washcloths on her face, rub her chest with my knuckles, jostle her while she was nursing, anything I could think of. Once she started taking full feedings, the snacking stopped and she would go 3-4 hours between meals. Even better, she was sleeping through the night by 12 weeks!

Leslie's Story: Living the Lifestyle

My Background

I am eight years older than my only sibling. I remember my mother nursing him, going to LLL meetings, and how great it was for them to have quiet time together. I grew up thinking babies are breastfed until they are ready to self wean (2-3 years old). I was shocked to find that most of my friends were not going to even try to breastfeed, and even ones that did might only try for a few weeks. I think moms are missing out on something wonderful. It is awesome to be able to comfort your baby this way, help them sleep, provide the best nutrition for them, and do it while relaxing!

Postpartum

We are creatures of hormones. All of our logical, rationale thoughts still come down to connections in the brain that are controlled by hormones. Postpartum can be really tough. The hormones that help maintain pregnancy come to a screeching halt and we are not only dealing with lack of sleep, a new baby and a new way of life, but hormones. Breastfeeding helps to regulate these hormones. When you letdown, you get a big dose of oxytocin (the love hormone). This helps you to bond with your baby and calms you down! It is one of the best ways to relax after a stressful day/night.

Some Pain

My daughter latched on within an hour of her natural childbirth (yep, no meds). She took to it like a fish to water. We never had any latch issues or concerns about her getting enough. Still, my nipples were tender. It didn't hurt to nurse except for the initial five seconds—OUCH! I would grind my teeth, clench my jaw and brace for the pain. But really within a few seconds it would be over and I would then try to relax my jaw and body while she nursed. This only lasted a week or two, and then once my nipples stretched out and toughened up there was no more pain. Once you get through the first few weeks, the hard part is over.

Letdown

I remember when I started to feel the letdowns; it was like ZING! Of course, if that happened when she wasn't nursing, it was like I could feel my breasts swelling! So I started to have to wear nursing pads. I couldn't use the cloth ones; I'd soak them in minutes. I had to use the disposable ones, and I like Lansinoh® the best. Some of the other ones had a smell to them. I can use the cloth ones now, but it took me 9-10 months before I could.

Sleep

I love to sleep. I love napping and getting up late! This was a big concern for me while I was pregnant. How on earth was I going to get sleep! Nighttime can be really hard for new moms. Babies have to eat often (every 2-4 hours), and they don't yet know that nighttime is for sleeping. I really think nursing and co-sleeping helped me get through the first few months and I know I got lots more sleep than my non-co-sleeping friends. I often say that I can handle almost anything after some sleep! Well-rested moms make much better moms!

When she would wake up at night to nurse, I was right there. I could get her nursing, and we could both fall asleep while she drank. There were times in the night that my daughter would wake to nurse and my husband would put her on me, and I didn't even wake up enough to notice. I used a puddle pad on the bed for several reasons: to catch any diaper leaks, spit ups, and me leaking. There are even studies out now to show that co-sleeping is safer and better for babies!

Now there were some nights that she just didn't want to sleep. At those times she would swing with the hairdryer on! I could catch a few winks on the couch while she swung. Once she got her days and nights straight, we could easily get a good solid 6-8 hours.

Lifestyle

I remember asking my mom about breastfeeding and she would always say, "It's a mothering style." I didn't get it until I became a breastfeeding mother myself. It is a mothering style, and I think a much easier style than bottle feeding. I have lots of girlfriends that bottle feed and most of their complaints are about sleeping. I really don't have any issues with sleeping. Naps are super easy, too. Just nurse and then there is a magic 7-10 minute window where you can put them down without waking them up! When she was little, I would just hold her. Trying to put her down could be tricky, but as she got older (3-4 months) it got easier. Even now as an 11-month-old, if she wakes up 30 minutes into the nap, I can go in and nurse her back to sleep.

I am an engineering, type A personality. I love schedules and routines, but babies bring about constant change! I am a much more relaxed mother because I breastfeed. Breastfeeding helps me go with the flow and to enjoy each moment and each phase (they change so quickly). I can be in the present because I'm not worrying about how to get her to nap or how many ounces she had today or what she did or didn't eat.

Nursing is a way of life that I highly recommend. But it does have a price. I can't consume anything I feel like. Foods have not affected my daughter, but what I drink sure does. I was on a lemonade kick—drinking about 2-3 glasses for several days—until I noticed she had developed diaper rash. I stopped drinking the lemonade, and the rash was gone. Almost any alcohol will get her fussy, too, and I do have to plan my wardrobe in advance if we are going to be out all day so I can nurse. All the advantages definitely outweigh these small disadvantages.

Nursing Tanks

I live in these. A girlfriend of mine gave me two, and I found them to be the most convenient for nursing, day or night. They hold the pads in place, I don't have to lift my shirt, and my tummy stays covered up while I nurse. My only issue came during wintertime when my shoulders would get cold; but I would wear my hoodies to bed or I had a lightweight robe.

Losing Weight

Let me just put it out there. I gained 60 pounds while pregnant. That is a lot of weight! I really thought I was doing good—only putting on five pounds the first trimester, but then by the third trimester I was packing on the pounds. I followed the Bradley Diet and was trying to get 80-100 grams of protein in a day. I was eating well, but maybe I had too much ice cream. (Next time around I'm going to lay off the ice cream.) Even with all that weight gain, after ten months postpartum I was back to within five pounds of my pre-pregnancy weight. I wasn't exercising or dieting like crazy, just eating healthy and running after my kid. So I'm here to tell you, the weight does come off and breastfeeding helps! You have to eat when breastfeeding, and if you don't, your body will tell you. Weight-watchers recommends 500 more calories a day, and you get it by two servings of fruit and milk. But honestly, during life changes I CRAVE chocolate, so I did have my share of brownies, and the weight still came off!

Healthy

This is a huge worry off my mind. I have girlfriends that have sick kids all the time. I know that my baby is getting antibodies from nursing, and let me tell you, we just aren't sick. We've only gotten two colds in 11 months.

Food

Around six months I started to expose my daughter to solid foods. She was so not interested. The advice I'd get from LLL mothers was that she will let you know when she is interested. I kept giving her things we were eating, and she would just spit them out. She was still gaining weight and nursing well, so I wasn't too worried. At 11 months (to the day!) she ate. I mean she chowed down a whole quesadilla! Now I have to remember to pack a snack for her; but really, nursing is still her main source of nourishment, and it's nice not having to worry about how much she is getting.

Teething

Around three months, she started to experiment. She was nipping at me when she wasn't super hungry. So I stopped trying to nurse her if she wasn't really ready to eat. At this time I found if I put my hand near her face (ready to detach at the first sign of biting) she was a more polite nurser. Luckily (like most things) this changed quickly, and after a week or so the experimentation stopped. Then the real teething began for us at seven months, and she would bite because her gums hurt. I would firmly set her on the floor and tell her "no bite." She would cry a little, and I would pick her up but not nurse again for several minutes. Even at eleven months (and six teeth later) she would still sometimes nip at me. When she did, I would sit her down and tell her "no bite." But this was a rare occurrence and is really not an issue.

Toddler Time

I think toddlers need to nurse. As long as you, your kid, and husband are okay with it, you should keep it up! At 19 months old, we still co-slept. This worked great for us. She slept and nursed throughout the night. I got GREAT sleep because I didn't have to wake up to settle a crying toddler.

Toddlers are going through HUGE changes and often they have meltdowns because they don't have the vocabulary or emotional intelligence to calmly explain their complex feelings. Nursing really helps them feel loved and calms them down. (The hormones released help Mommy to calm down, too!)

Kids need to suck. It is built into our DNA and nursing provides a good outlet for that. Nursing allows them to suck and lets their mouth develop properly. If you are not nursing your toddler, then they might take to sucking things that could harm their mouth development.

There have been studies that also show the size of your baby's brain can be determined by how long they nurse. The average weaning age across the world is 4.6 years. The emperors of China were nursed until they were eight. Our immune system is not fully functional until six years old. I'm not saying I will nurse my child that long, but we will nurse until we are ready to wean and will not be swayed by a bottle-fed society.

Support Groups

I go to LLL meetings. It's kind of funny how much I don't have in common with the women at LLL except for how we raise our children. I go to hear advice from other breastfeeding mothers. It's so nice to feel like what you are doing isn't crazy, that it is what the majority of mothers do around the world and it is best. Before I was a mother, I used to think it was weird how moms would just whip out their boobs and kids would drink. I think our society has sexualized breasts. But now that I am a nursing mother, I can tell you there is nothing weird about it. It is comforting and provides a closeness that can only be found through nursing. Because of this aspect of our relationship, I am more in tuned to my daughter and her needs.

Gwen's Story: No Mom is an Island

As a new mom, I cannot emphasize enough the need for a support system while breastfeeding. If it had not been for my husband, family, friends, and lactation consultants, I would have quit the first week. Standard breastfeeding challenges were made greater by the fact that my little girl was born five weeks early. She spent six days in the nursery—I never had her in the room with me. She was able to suck on her own, but her mouth was so tiny that she couldn't get a good latch. Due to that and because she was in the nursery, she had formula in a bottle the first 4 days of life until my milk came in. I am a true testament that babies can exclusively breastfeed even if they've been given formula or a bottle in the hospital!

I asked for a lactation consultant at the hospital at least one feeding per day—more if they were available—to help us get a good latch. The hospital is your best opportunity to get help, so be demanding!! At the beginning of each feeding, even before my milk came in, we would try to nurse for about 10 minutes or less—just before she got too frustrated—then we would go to the bottle. Once we brought her home, she was still struggling with the latch, so we fed her pumped breast milk from a bottle. Her gag reflex was not fully developed yet, though, so she choked a lot. This was very upsetting!

After a week at home, I went to our local breastfeeding resource center for help. They recommended I try a nipple shield so she could control the flow instead of the bottle nipple. That worked wonders! I was able to breastfeed instead of pump, and my daughter adapted well to the nipple shield. It was a little messy because the milk would collect in the shield faster than she drank, but I just always used a burp cloth under her neck. We were also able to nurse in public using the shield. It did take some practice to get good at maneuvering, but we conquered it. Each one of these little milestones was empowering. After a couple months of using the shield, I began to try nursing her naturally. It only took a couple days for her to adapt without the shield. I was so proud of her ability and my patience!

As I said above, none of this would have been possible without my support system. My husband would get up early after she ate and let me sleep. I felt lazy sleeping until 10am, but I wouldn't have been functional otherwise. He went with me to the breastfeeding classes prior to birth and to the breastfeeding resource center when I needed help. My family and friends were very understanding even though they weren't that familiar with breastfeeding. If we were out, they were willing to stop what we were doing so I could nurse. Whoever was with me would help me get settled and hold the baby while I got situated to switch sides. I had to explain how some things worked and why she ate so often, but once they knew, it was never an issue. I was in an out-of-town wedding three months after baby was born and my best friend even arranged the day so I would have breaks to pump!

Knowing I would eventually go back to work, we started giving our baby one bottle a day when she was six weeks old. We waited a little longer than some because she was a preemie. I went back to work three months after giving birth and my little one went to a daycare center. I pumped at work every three hours. I encourage you to make sure your caregiver knows the proper way to handle breast milk—many don't! I won't say it wasn't difficult, but once I got in the routine it went very smoothly. I blocked the time off on my calendar so no one could schedule meetings when I had to pump. It was a way to connect to her during the day and take time out to think about being a mom. In Illinois it is a state law that employers have to provide a private place to pump—and not in a bathroom. I am not sure how many states are like that, but if your employer resists, don't give up. You are feeding your baby—no one should deny you that right. At night and on the weekends, I exclusively breastfed unless we wanted a few hours away.

Attitude is also a big part of it—you can't be worried too much about what others think when you're nursing in public or making decisions about how to raise your baby. I am one that reads all I can about a subject, but there are so many differing opinions that it can be overwhelming. I had to learn to trust my instincts and do what was best for us. Take advice with a grain of salt—in most situations there are several 'right ways' of doing it!

Stories of
Confidence

A feeling or consciousness of one's powers or of reliance on one's circumstances.

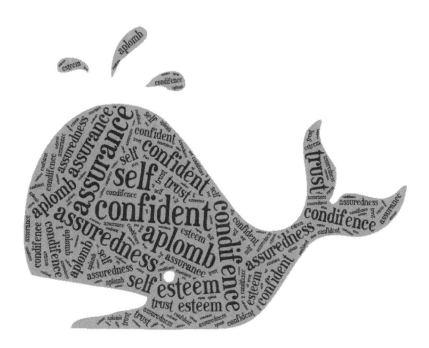

Zoë's Story: Preemie Power

The birth and first few months with my first child was nothing like I had planned. I had intended to have a natural birth with no drugs and breastfeed in the birthing room. I'd read about breastfeeding, taken the breastfeeding class, and was dead set on nursing.

This was all challenged when I was admitted to the hospital in my third trimester and put on bed rest with 24/7 monitoring. The baby was in danger and "any day could be the day," so I was in the Labor and Delivery unit ready to go for 3 weeks. It was very stressful. And when the high risk doctors decided that the risks outweighed the benefits of him still being en utero, he was delivered early via C-section without me ever having gone into labor.

I got to see him, but he was quickly taken away for monitoring and then later taken to the NICU Level 4. It was another 24 hours before I got to see him and six days before I got to hold him. In fact, I had to leave the hospital without ever having held my new baby. It was heart breaking! So, as you can imagine, none of the natural physical bonding took place. I could not nuzzle with him, since I could not even hold him. I started pumping straight away, but my body had never gone into labor and it had been a very stressful three weeks on hospitalized bed rest. The nurses sent up blankets of his for me to smell to try to stimulate my milk production, but that didn't help and made me feel more upset. It was definitely not a good start to our nursing relationship. I had nurses and others tell me to give up on nursing, get some rest, and focus on getting myself better from surgery and bed rest.

But I was still determined to nurse him. I was pumping eight times a day, although weakened from the weeks on bed rest and the C-section. When I did get to see him, they said he was too weak to try to put him to my breast, so I did "kangaroo care" and just held him skin to skin for an hour a day—that's all they would let me do. I tried the herbal supplements and prescription Reglan. I felt like I tried every tip anyone gave me. And when I was allowed to try nursing for the first time, my little one wouldn't latch on. And when he did at last, he was so weak he didn't suck very hard. It was frustrating for all involved! And I was sad, because I so wanted to breastfeed. Any little drop I did get, the nurses put in his feeding tube and then later into bottles, so that gave me some satisfaction.

But my story has a happy ending! We stuck with it and we succeeded! At first, I was only allowed to nurse him once a day so he didn't get too tired (bottles are easier on babies and take less effort). But eventually, we were nursing several times a day and went on to do so until he was 13 months old! My body never did produce enough milk for him so he was always supplemented with formula; but every ounce I ever made, he got. We treated it like liquid gold in our house! But we had the experience, and he got the benefits in the end.

With my second child, it was an entirely different. It was much more of what I had expected and longed for the first time around. We nursed in the recovery room after my repeat C-section and, in fact, we went on to nurse for 18 months and she never had a drop of formula. This pleased me in the sense of, "my body CAN do it after all!" I am now positive it was the stress of the situation with my first child that affected my milk production. I am very grateful to have had an easier go with my second baby, but it makes me even more proud that I didn't throw in the towel with my first child.

So my message to all mothers is that you CAN do it as long as you really want to and you have perseverance. Perhaps the biggest thing is to have the confidence that you CAN do it, because especially after an experience like the NICU where nurses and doctors are taking care of your baby around the clock, you are at risk of losing the confidence that you are this baby's mother. But you are exactly what he needs. I hope my story helps in the sense that even the roughest starts can turn out great in the end.

Tips

- Have a buddy that you can call day or night when things are not going well. Husbands are wonderful, but they don't understand like another nursing mother does.

- I had to use a nipple shield with both kiddos because, apparently, the drugs from the C-sections made my nipples flat and therefore they had trouble latching on.

- I never used both breasts in one feeding. I always did one full side per feeding.

- Preemies nurse longer than full term babies. Many people told me that I was letting him nurse too long and that he was using me only for comfort. I read recently in a LLL publication that preemies take longer because they are smaller and weaker. I wish I'd let him suckle more. I think that would have helped with my milk production.

- Use the cotton breast pads! They get so soft after a few washes and hold up well for subsequent babies.

- If your baby is having trouble digesting foods, don't give up nursing! With both of my babies I had to really change my diet (ie: no dairy, no gluten) for many months. But my view was that I'd do anything for my child and that this was one season of my life, so why wouldn't I? You'd be amazed at what alternatives are out there (ie: gluten free pasta and bread, soy cheese, and chocolate pudding).

- I also found that giving the Mylicon® Infant Gas Drops before a feeding worked better for my kids than giving it after as per the instructions. I did check with the NICU nurse on this, but I'd advise you to double check as well.

- We LOVED our Boppy® pillow. Not only did it help prop up baby for a good position, it also protected my C-section wound from being kicked.

- If your baby bites, just take them off the breast and say "no" once and put them on a blanket on the floor. You should only have to do this once or twice, as they learn quickly that biting will result in losing not only the milk but mommy's affection, too!

- Going back to my story above, I pumped so much with my first baby that I burned out the motor on my pump. So, for the second baby I got the much better one (the $250 one) and it was a hundred times better. I wished I'd just bought that one in the first place.

- My second child showed no signs of wanting to stop nursing. I think it would have gone on forever had I not weaned her at 18 months. By this point it was only before nap and before bedtime, so to make it that much easier my husband started putting her to bed and then she wasn't looking to nurse. Within a few days, we were done and that was that. I think that babies get into routines and at least for me, I felt like changing a certain routine would be horrible. Chances are, they'll adapt to the one change just fine when everything else stays the same. I think she was ready, but I don't think she knew otherwise because she never would accept a bottle. We had to go straight to sippy cups, and I found that the ones with straws were much easier for her to understand.

Don't think that you have to feel "done" with nursing to end that chapter. It's been a year since I nursed and I still miss it. I have dreams about it from time to time even. It was a wonderful, joyous experience once we got over the initial weeks (or months with my first born). I was so glad that I nursed my children. I have zero regrets.

K.C.'s Story:
Breast is Best

Breastfeeding is often no walk in the park for a first-time mom. My experience was painful both physically and emotionally. But don't let my story scare you; my case was pretty extreme.

After trying to conceive for over three years, my husband and I finally discovered we were pregnant. Pregnancy was an unexpected blessing, so we took nothing for granted those nine months. We only bought organic. I swore off caffeine, deli meat, and sushi. I took my vitamins daily, and we never missed a doctor's appointment.

As a soon-to-be parent, the message was everywhere I turned, *"Breast is best."* In my quest for the best, I waddled into a breastfeeding class a few weeks prior to my due date. I went alone because the topic was squeamish enough for me, let alone my husband. As it happened, there was one guy in attendance. I would be lying if I said I wasn't a bit miffed about that at the time. (Now I realize it was no big deal. Sure, there were some birthing videos and candid shots of women's leaking breasts, but dads have to be prepared, too, right? Poor fella.)

Anyway, we get to the Q&A portion and several women start asking why their breasts were leaking. *Say what? I didn't have that problem.* This was the first indication that I wasn't like everyone else, but I shrugged it off.

Two weeks after my class, I gave birth to a healthy baby girl! The delivery was, let's just say, *messy.* I had third degree tearing that earned me a bunch of stitches. I was pumped full of drugs, so my memory has grown a bit fuzzy, but I can tell you she wasn't laid on my chest to root at my breast like the stuff I saw on TV. Instead, I was given a brief moment to hold her and then she was whisked out of the room with my husband in tow. Apparently the doctor needed time to figure out how to put me back together again.

After regaining my senses, I found myself in a hospital room with a baby sleeping peacefully in a cart next to my bed. Then it hit me, *Um, I should probably feed her. Oh, dear. What was it that lady said in class?* I starting flipping frantically through the breastfeeding handouts I brought with me to the hospital. After a quick prep for my pop quiz, my husband handed her to me. She was still sound asleep. *Ah, yes, the baby may want to sleep through a feeding. Get a wet cloth to rub on her feet. No wait—undress her so the cool air wakes her, or was it…?* I was totally clueless.

After several maneuvers to rouse her from sleep, she finally woke up enough for me to attempt a latch. Keyword being "attempt" because it was a total fail. She couldn't latch, wouldn't latch. I was so dry my kid must have tasted dust. I had no leaky breasts, *nothing.* When I finally got her to semi-latch, she would suck fruitlessly—leaving my breast raw with each attempt.

I don't even remember how long it was before we called in the lactation consultant. She was a sturdy, no-nonsense kind of woman who grabbed my baby's head like a ragdoll and rammed her face into my breast repeatedly. We tried this exercise for about ten minutes until she finally proclaimed that I had to keep practicing and, in time, my milk would come in. Then off she went.

Now what? Give my kid the evil poison? The thought left me feeling hopeless and awful. My baby was not even on this earth for 24 hours and I had already failed her.

We called in one of the nurses on duty and asked her opinion as to what we should do next. *How much formula could we give her? How long could we bottle-feed without making her refuse to nurse?* The nurse was very careful to sidestep the breastfeeding versus formula issue. All we got out of her was the recommended amount of formula per feeding. It was useless trying to ask her anything else, so we thanked her for her time and kept our litany of questions to ourselves.

Breast is best, but just this once, I thought, staring at a bottle of formula. After all, my baby needs to eat. Just this once and then I'll figure it all out.

Shortly after giving her the bottle, we were both resting peacefully when I noticed she spat most of her milk back up. I was scared out of my mind, so I called the hospital pediatrician. He was not too pleased to hear that I was having trouble nursing. *"Why didn't you call me first?"*

201

After giving me a proper scolding, the pediatrician explained how to supplement: 20 minutes on one breast, 20 minutes on the other, and then a half-serving of formula to top her off.

My daughter spat up profusely after each feeding, but a nurse reassured us that spitting up was normal.

We were discharged from the hospital, but shortly after getting home, we noticed that she was growing more orange by the hour. The chubby baby I gave birth to started to look sick and scrawny. After several hours of dry nursing attempts, we were exhausted and bewildered. We gave her some formula to "top her off," but she couldn't keep any of it down. We finally decided something was seriously wrong when she spat up most during a diaper change or when we placed her on her back. The combination of her inability to latch, her orange hue, and her constant spitting up landed us in the doctor's office within less than a day of taking her home.

The verdict? She had gastrointestinal reflux, lactose intolerance, and a borderline case of jaundice. *Well, if that didn't complicate things.* We were given a prescription with specific instructions on how to administer the medication: starting fifteen minutes before each feeding, we had to give my daughter her "syrup" for the reflux. Most of the time, she hated it and screamed bloody murder. After the syrup, we had to keep her upright for the fifteen minutes leading up to each feeding.

I was still attempting to nurse and continued the supplementing routine—alternating on each breast with a few ounces of formula to top her off. We had to keep her upright for 15 minutes following each feeding, too. Thankfully my husband helped when he could and would hold her upright while I fruitlessly tried to pump an ounce or so between feedings.

While conducting some research, I discovered a local women's center that offered paid lactation counseling. The price was steep, but after having limited success with breastfeeding, we decided the expense was worth it. I remember the lactation consultant's surprise when she learned of my dilemma. She glanced at my chest and said something along the lines of how bustier moms of my ethnicity (I'm part Hispanic) usually have no trouble producing milk. I didn't know whether to laugh or cry.

Overall she was quite helpful and compassionate, but there was only so much ground we could cover in one hour. We practiced a few nursing positions, then the session ended with a recommendation for a larger breast shield (go figure), and plenty of water. Busty as I am, I don't think I ever produced more than 3 ounces between each breast. Whatever milk I was able to produce was carefully stored in the freezer for my famous breast milk & formula cocktails.

After all, *breast is best.*

The first few months of parenthood were grueling. My baby brought a light into our lives that made the effort well worth it, but I can't say it was ever easy and those memories are mostly marked by pain. My breasts were scabbed and bleeding from the ill attempts at getting a good latch. I was sore from the delivery and the pain didn't subside until well after three months. Above all, I was heartbroken. I couldn't give her the *best*—no matter how hard I tried.

I drove myself crazy trying everything under the sun. Compresses, nipple guards, gel patches, herbal teas, beer (that part wasn't so bad), milk thistle, warm baths…you name it, I tried it. I owned everything made for breastfeeding, too. A top-of-the-line breast pump, nursing covers, breastfeeding tops, nursing bras, oh and don't forget the Boppy® pillow with the cute interchangeable cupcake-patterned cover.

Needless to say, I was exhausted all the time. *Sleep when your baby sleeps*, they said. While she slept, I was connected to a breast pump in the hopes of stimulating my milk supply. At one point, I chucked that breast pump across the room I felt so frustrated and defeated.

But I did it because *breast is best*.

I was the odd girl out, too. During my pregnancy, I was lucky to have two acquaintances (wives of my husband's coworkers) that were also expecting. They both already had one child apiece and were constantly swapping stories about breastfeeding, childrearing, etc. I listened intently; soaking up every word—knowing the time was soon coming for me to put all that advice into action.

When the time did come, while they were breastfeeding their kids with ease, I was shaking up a bottle of soy formula. And that's when the questions came, "How much do you pay for formula? Isn't it expensive?"

Breast is best.

For me, breastfeeding was also isolating. I belonged to the camp where you should nurse discreetly so as not to weird out the people around you. Once, I tried to play with the cool kids and donned a new nursing cover while awkwardly trying to feed my baby underneath. It was a humiliating experience because I couldn't produce any milk and I had to ditch my efforts in favor of a bottle. I'm sure they didn't mean to show pity, but it was plainly written on their faces.

When my daughter was about a month old, my sister and her boyfriend flew into town for a visit. I didn't get to spend much time with her because I was holed up in my room trying to nurse my baby. Thinking back about that makes me sad because I don't get to see her often and I totally missed the opportunity. Come to think of it, I missed out on a lot of opportunities for not facing facts.

Breast is best.

Or is it?

What I think is best is that you try to be a good parent while accepting your limitations. I wish I had accepted my own limitations sooner and stopped being so uptight. I would have been a better parent for it.

A friend of mine recently shared some advice that I want to pass along to anyone having trouble nursing. Set a reasonable time limit for yourself...long enough to know when it's time to hold 'em or fold 'em. Although I don't think moms should abandon breastfeeding for sake of convenience and sleep; there are those rare cases like mine where "breast isn't best" for various reasons. Women need to understand that there might be a larger picture involved to explain why another mom can't/won't breastfeed and not be so quick to judge.

Even good parents make mistakes along the way. I failed miserably at breastfeeding, but I didn't fail to try. I'm learning to find peace with that. If you find yourself in the same boat for whatever reason, I hope you will, too.

Jodie's Story: Patience is a Virtue

First things first: stop, step back, and take a big deep breath. In front of you is the most precious gift that you will ever receive in your entire life. I am a mother of three (two boys and a girl) and a stay-at-home mom who takes care of my friend's three children and my nephew. I nursed my sons until they were 14 months old. My daughter was only nursed until she was about 10 months old when we found out that we were pregnant with our third child. Reluctantly I quit but all was good. She managed just fine with milk and I survived also.

I found nursing to be quite a wonderful bonding time for me and the children. I never took a breastfeeding class and never really read too much information on it. I am not going to sit here and tell you that it is easy, or it doesn't hurt, or it isn't time consuming, because that would be a lie. But for me, formula was never an option.

There is a big time commitment when it comes to breastfeeding your child. Sometimes it is every couple hours, and sometimes it is every hour. There will be days when you don't get much done because the baby needs you. But you know what? That's ok. For some people that is a very hard thing to accept, that the schedule and routine that you were accustomed to is no longer your choice.

As you take your new child out and about, you are going to have to deal with trying to feed this very hungry baby in very unusual places. First off relax, because if you don't, your baby won't and feeding will not go well. Babies feed off of how mom is feeling.

Next, remember that God put your boobs on this earth to feed your children, and everything else that goes on with them is just a plus.

You are going to run into people that are put off by breastfeeding and others that are more than supportive of it. I was always one that would do it anywhere at any time in front of anyone. They have come out with a lot of things to keep you covered. As for me, I used a burp cloth and my shirt to cover me up and that was just easier for me, but you do what works best for you. Don't rush it; take your time. The more you do it, the easier and more discreet it will become.

That goes for breastfeeding in general. You can't go in expecting to be perfect from day one. You are learning, the baby is learning, and you will constantly be finding new ways to do it and make it easier for you and your baby.

Long story short, it is a wonderful thing that you can do for you and your child. However, it is not the easiest thing in the world. If it was, everyone would do it. Take your time, relax, and be patient. It will click in due time. Women have been doing it for thousands of years without the books, modern technology, and the frills. The books and videos are good as long as you don't take it word for word. Lean on your family and friends and get away from time to time; you need your time and space in order to be the best mother you can be. Everyone is going to give you ideas and suggestions and that is what they are—ideas and suggestions—not the law. Use your common sense, have fun, and congrats on your new bundle of joy.

Angie's Story: Keeping the Faith

Mini Me

When my second child was born, my oldest was 2½. My daughter always sat with me while I nursed her baby brother. One day as I settled down to nurse, she came out of her room with a baby doll. She sat down at my feet, pulled up her shirt and pressed her baby doll to her chest. She sat there like that the entire time I nursed and even switched sides! As I watched her then I wondered if she would mimic me on other things. Now, as she is about to enter middle school, I can see how she has copied my actions and behaviors on so many things, just as she did back then nursing her baby doll. And please note, especially if this is your first child or your children are very young, those precious babies copy *everything* you do as they grow up—good and bad!

A Note about Weaning and Worry

I worried a lot about weaning with my first baby. As one year of nursing came to a close, I had no idea how to cut it off. One day, there simply was no milk. My daughter didn't even notice! It was as simple as that. With each of the next three babies, I tried to relax about weaning and eventually I dried up and the milk was gone. With my last baby (and honestly I was in no hurry to end then), I was still nursing him to sleep at night at 15 months. One night he fell asleep before I could nurse him. The next night he wasn't interested. The following day the milk was gone and we were done with nursing.

Weaning was a true example to me that worry is wasted time. It reminds me of the phrase "let go and let God." Nursing is such a perfect system and your body gets so in tune with the baby. Just relax and let things go as they should go—and don't let anyone pressure and worry you to do otherwise.

God said it best: So don't worry about these things, saying, 'What will we eat? What will we drink? What will we wear?' These things dominate the thoughts of unbelievers, but your heavenly Father already knows all your needs. Seek the Kingdom of God above all else, and live righteously, and he will give you everything you need. (Matthew 6:31-33, NLT).

Susan's Story: The Juggling Act

Trying to juggle staying fit and being a nursing mom is definitely a challenge. I managed to stay in pretty decent shape throughout both of my pregnancies, and wanted to keep it up after my second baby was born. Easier said than done! Besides being completely exhausted keeping up with my 3-year old, I now had a newborn to tend to. I planned to nurse my second child for 12 months (and exclusively for the first 6 months) like I did my first, but I knew that it would be beneficial for everyone if I kept up my workouts, too. (I tend to get a little crabby if I don't get some "me" time. Oh yeah, and I also like to eat. Surely exercising and nursing a baby justifies at least one generous bowl of ice cream at night? I think so!)

So after my 6-week checkup, I decided to start training for a half marathon. I had six months to get in shape, and I had not run since my first trimester. I prepared for the challenges ahead through seeking balance, sleep, and a very supportive bra!

So where to begin? I figured out right away that I would need to feed baby before running. Trying to run loaded down with milk is extremely uncomfortable. I would also need to double up on sports bras; there was no getting around that. There was also the question of time. When was I supposed to find time to exercise? Just trying to get ready for a run was exhausting enough: first I would feed the baby, then layer up my sports bras, warm up, give my husband instructions, and lastly make sure my three year old was content. I was ready for a nap before my run even began!

On days when I was doing my long runs, I would usually drive to a nearby park. And since I am by no means a fast runner, it would usually turn into an all-day event. There is nothing like coming home all sweaty and exhausted to a crying infant needing to be fed again and a husband standing there looking helpless! Did I mention my baby doesn't like to take a bottle? Yeah, things definitely got easier when she turned 6 months and we started her on solids.

Throughout my training I found that running first thing in the morning was best—although maybe not easiest. I am not a morning person to begin with; then add to the equation a baby that doesn't sleep through the night, and I was really not feeling like lacing up the sneakers. But trying to squeeze a run in any other time of the day was tough. Plus it was nice to get it over with and come back to a quiet house and enjoy my coffee while everyone was still sleeping! The main challenge of morning workouts was that I either needed to feed the baby or pump first, or triple up the sports bra. Fun times!

Race day came and went, and it was a success! I was able to finish in the time that I was hoping for, even though baby dear decided to stay up until midnight the night before. I even had to allow enough time to pump before I left for the race, so I was running on adrenaline and not much else!

I really felt that training for something outside of breastfeeding and having a goal to work towards really helped my whole experience. Having a weekly plan helped me see what I had to fit in, too. I didn't always stick to it, but I usually came pretty close. I opted for the bare bones training so I wasn't overwhelmed and even found a plan where I only had to run a total of 3-4 times a week.

I learned a lot through this experience, like how not to set unreasonable goals for myself and to remember I can only do so much! It is all about time management, a lot of rest, hydration, and a very understanding spouse. I came up with every excuse in the book not to get out of bed in the morning, but I always managed to anyway. Find what makes you happy and do it! I just signed up for a sprint triathlon. Now to find time for swimming, biking, and running. Hmmm…

Sarah's Story: Keep Calm and Carry On

My motto for breastfeeding was to do it only as long as it worked for baby and me. My sister had tons of issues, most of which were brought about (in my opinion) by overthinking and overcomplicating what can be a very natural process. That said, I know I had a really easy time with nursing and some just don't have that. Anyway, that "as long as it works" attitude helped me feel less pressure going into nursing. I never felt that if I had to quit it would have been a huge issue, and I'm convinced that this attitude helped me relax about the whole thing. (Incidentally, my sister gave up three weeks into nursing and felt that was the best decision she ever made. I supported her fully after the ordeal she endured getting to that decision.)

Mastitis

For as relatively easy as nursing was, I had mastitis once with Ann. The substitute on-call doctor tried to tell me I had the flu. What kind of flu comes on in an hour, turns one breast bright red and hurts like crazy, creates a breast that pumps puss and blood instead of milk (while the other is completely normal) and makes it so uncomfortable to pump that you throw up from the pain? As a new mom and unsure as I was, I just took

Johnson's Tylenol® and tried to take it easy. By the next night, I was too weak to lift Ann to the good side. Finally we went to the ER where they gave me IV antibiotics and fluids to get the infection under control. If that doctor had put me on antibiotics right away, we would have probably avoided the whole emergency room thing and a bunch of anguish altogether!

With Lauren, I had mastitis on the left side more times than I can remember (a case of meningitis prior to pregnancy made everything much more difficult for the second time around). After countless rounds of Augmentin and Dycolxicillin, my OB/GYN sent me to a surgeon to have the breast infection drained, and they ended up removing the most gnarly and twisted mammary duct. Through the whole thing, though, I kept nursing (dumping the nasty left side and feeding from the right). Surgery was an instant fix, and I felt so great the night of the surgery that I went home and cooked dinner!

Mastitis is the most awful thing to endure. Words of advice if you have it: get on an antibiotic IMMEDIATELY as it festers and worsens into the most heinous "flu" you can fathom; keep nursing/pumping to work the infection out and keep the plumbing lines as clear as possible; use moist heat (shower, warm washcloth, or a moist heating pad); and express/pump/nurse as often as you can stand it.

Bound and Determined

Ann was 3½ and Lauren was just a few weeks old. My husband was out of town, and we had one of those absolutely amazing spring days. Ann wanted to ride her bike, but it was one of those big wheels with the parent push-handle in the back. We only made it around the cul de sac once before I realized this was an entirely futile effort. With no way to push a stroller and this crazy contraption of hers, I headed off to Toys R Us to get the tricycle we had promised her and just hadn't purchased yet. Frugal and feminist, I declined the $10 assembly and decided to assemble on my own. As the afternoon hours turned toward evening, a rather impatient 3 ½ year old just HAD to go for a ride at the exact same time Lauren HAD to eat. Not willing to be beaten by circumstance, I balanced Lauren on my knee and nursed her WHILE assembling the tricycle on the back patio. I don't think my neighbors knew WHAT was going on. I was completely proud of my maternal multitasking! We made it out in time for a splendid trike ride and baby stroll, and the tricycle remains the most solidly assembled piece of equipment in the garage!

When You Gotta Nurse, You Gotta Nurse

The most memorable place my baby was fed would have to be in the luggage/check-in line at the airport in Maui. Too many tour groups hit the airport at one time and we wouldn't have made our flight if I hadn't stood in line. We were so inconspicuous that my own husband didn't even know what Ann was up to!

Mindy's Story: Independence Day

July 4, 2008 found me and my family celebrating in the parking lot of our church. I adore the 4th of July with all its pomp and pageantry, a gorgeous cornucopia of colors exploding from flagpoles and the midnight sky. And I love the perceived feeling of unification across the country. For a day, we can all relish hot dogs and civil liberties and homemade ice cream and the right to speak our minds.

This particular holiday, we were a state away from our families. Seeing that it fell in the middle of the week, we chose not to drive the eight hours to hometown "Mayberry." Actually, our church allows members and guests to park in the lot and watch the fireworks bursting overhead at the nearby park. In the waning heat of the day and the buildup of anticipation, members provide an old-fashioned "Music Man" homage—with barbershop quartets and fresh popcorn interspersed with gospel.

My husband and I eagerly toted our three-year old and six-month old along to celebrate the nation's birthday with other like-minded folk. Night soon came and before the start of the explosive luminaries, my baby was hungry. Not wanting to offend anyone's delicate sensibilities, I retreated to the car to feed him. We were parked far in the back of the filled lot, and with darkness settling, I decided to forgo the receiving blanket over my little guy's head. A gentle, cool summer breeze washed over us as I reclined in the front and relaxed while he nursed quietly.

Our sweet tableau was disturbed by a passing rush of haughty air, followed by the intrusive words, "Disgusting! She should cover up!" A middle-aged couple had passed by the car—the man turning back for what I can only guess was another gander. They were indignant, like a dog had just marked its territory on their lawn. (In all fairness, I could have covered up since we were in public. But the most offensive part was their attitude towards my choice of feeding.)

Prior to that evening I had fed in a Porta-Potty and various bathroom stalls—filthy, germ-infested hovels. This was much more appealing to my baby, I am sure! I knew how fortunate I was, too, since there are many women who cannot nurse for various reasons. So, knowing full well that breastfeeding in public is a protected right, I went right on nursing—smugly pleased that my simple action of mothering had caused such a reaction from "the establishment."

For every glare and provocative comment aimed at a nursing mom, there are four moms behind her saying, "Hey, would you rather hear a crying baby?!" And of all days, on Independence Day we should celebrate our chapped red nipples, blue veins, and white bosoms...because somewhere a future president is switching sides.

Bibliography

"Breast Milk Storage Guidelines." (Online)
http://www.justmommies.com/articles/breast-milk-
storage.shtml (visited: February 8, 2012).

"Breast milk Storage & Handling." (Online)
http://kellymom.com/bf/pumpingmoms/milkstorage/milkstorag
e/#storage (visited: February 8, 2012).

Colburn-Smith, Cate, and Andrea Serrette. The Milk Memos:
How Real Moms Learned to Mix Business with Babies-and
How You Can, Too. Tarcher. 2007.

Ezzo, Gary, and Robert Bucknam. On Becoming Baby Wise:
Giving Your Infant the GIFT of Nighttime Sleep. Parent-Wise
Solutions. 2012.

Ferber, Richard. Solve Your Child's Sleep Problems: New,
Revised, and Expanded Edition. Touchstone. 2006.

Hale, Thomas W., Medications and Mothers' Milk: A Manual
of Lactational Pharmacology. Pharmasoft Medical Pub. 2004.

Hicks, Jennifer. Hirkani's Daughters: Women Who Scale
Modern Mountains to Combine Breastfeeding and Working. La
Leche League International. 2005.

Hogg, Tracy, and Melinda Blau. Secrets of the Baby Whisperer: How to Calm, Connect, and Communicate with Your Baby. Ballantine Books. 2005.

Holy Bible Text Edition New Living Translation. Tyndale House Publishers. 2004.

Huggins, Kathleen. The Nursing Mother's Companion, 6th Edition: 25th Anniversary Edition. Harvard Common Press. 2010.

Karp, Harvey. The Happiest Baby on the Block. Bantam. 2003.

Pantley, Elizabeth. The No-Cry Sleep Solution: Gentle Ways to Help Your Baby Sleep Through the Night. McGraw-Hill. 2002.

Pryor, Gale, and Kathleen Huggins. Nursing Mother, Working Mother, Revised Edition. The Harvard Common Press. 2007.

Sears, William, and Mary Sears. The Attachment Parenting Book: A Commonsense Guide to Understanding and Nurturing Your Baby. Little, Brown and Company. 2001.

Sears, William, and Mary Sears. The Fussy Baby Book: Parenting Your High-Need Child From Birth to Age Five. Little, Brown and Company. 1996.

Steiner, Andy. Spilled Milk: Breastfeeding Adventures and Advice from Less-Than Perfect Moms. Rodale Books. 2005.

Tamaro, Janet. So That's What They're For!: The Definitive Breastfeeding Guide 3rd edition. 2005.

"The Transfer of Drugs and Other Chemicals Into Human Milk."(Online) http://pediatrics.aappublications.org/content/ 108/3/776.full.pdf+html. *Pediatrics*. 2001. (visited June 20, 2012).

"Water Conservation Facts and Tips." (Online) http://www.sscwd.org/tips.html (visited: February 8, 2012).

Weissbluth, Marc. Healthy Sleep Habits, Happy Child. Ballantine Books. 1999.

Wendkos Olds, Sally, and Laura Marks. The Complete Book of Breastfeeding, 4th edition: The Classic Guide. Workman Publishing Company. 2010.

West, Diana, and Lisa Marasco. The Breastfeeding Mother's Guide to Making More Milk. McGraw-Hill. 2008.

Wiessinger, Diane, Diana West, and Teresa Pitman. The Womanly Art of Breastfeeding. Ballantine Books. 2010.

Glossary

AAP The American Academy of Pediatrics (AAP) is "an organization of 60,000 physicians committed to the optimal physical, mental, and social health and well-being for all infants, children, adolescents, and young adults."

Bradley Diet A natural diet created for optimum pregnancy and health. See http://www.bradleybirth.com/Diet.aspx for more information.

Breast Shield Also called a nipple shield, this cap or dome (with an opening in the center from which baby nurses) goes over the nipple and areola to allow the flow of milk, provide a larger surface for the baby to latch onto, and protect the breast if they are sore.

Colic When a healthy, well-fed baby who is not in pain cries or shows symptoms of distress for extended periods of time without discernable reason. Bouts of (often inconsolable) crying usually last more than 1-2 hours (a stricter rule of thumb defines colic as lasting more than 3 hours a day for more than 3 days a week for more than 3 weeks.) The condition usually begins 2-4 weeks after birth and ends by the third month of life—peaking around six weeks of age. Some colicky babies respond to being held and shhhhed; others respond well to white noise. See the Happiest Baby on the Block by Harvey Karp for more tips. Although tempting, do not drive a colicky baby around in the car to help her sleep while you are tired!

Colostrum The yellowish breast milk produced the first few days after birth before you "milk comes in." This nutrient-rich substance is full of antibodies to boost baby's immune system.

D&C Dilation and curettage (D&C) refers to a surgical procedure in which the cervix is dilated and a special instrument is used to scrape the uterine lining. Anesthesia is used during the procedure and recovery time is generally short. Cramping and light bleeding may occur.

E.A.S.Y. A system developed by the late Tracy Hogg to help create structure for mom and baby: E stands for *eat*; A stand for *activity* (such as lullabies, bath time, toys, diaper changes, time with visitors, etc.); S stands for *sleep* (ranging from 20 minutes to 2 hours as baby grows and develops); and Y stands for *you* (a time to recharge with a cat nap, bath, a good book, etc. before baby rouses). See Secrets of the Baby Whisperer for more information.

Ferber Method Richard Ferber's method begins with a warm, loving bedtime routine and ends with putting your child in bed awake and leaving him (even if he cries) for gradually longer periods of time. This teaches baby how to self-soothe.

Food Trial As opposed to simply avoiding certain foods like coffee or dairy that may affect baby, a food trial (sometimes called an elimination diet) goes a step further by only eating certain foods and gradually adding others back. There's an in-depth explanation on the Ask Dr. Sears site at http://www.askdrsears.com/topics/feeding-infants-toddlers/food-allergies/elimination-diet.

Foremilk The milk that first comes out during a feeding. It is thinner and lower in calories—mainly serves to quench baby's thirst.

Hindmilk The milk which follows foremilk during a feeding which is thicker, creamier, and contains higher levels of fat and calories. It's important to "empty" one breast before moving to the other to ensure baby reaps the nutritional value.

Jaundice Newborn jaundice (physiologic jaundice) occurs in many babies. It becomes cause for concern when bilirubin levels reach dangerous levels (which can cause brain damage). You're encouraged to nurse often because bilirubin will recirculate in the body until it is excreted in baby's stool. Colostrum acts as a laxative to push it out (thus reducing bilirubin levels).

Kangaroo Care Named for its similarity with how mother kangaroos care for their young, this technique involves holding (often premature) newborn babies skin-to-skin—usually his mother and/or father—to ensure physiological and psychological closeness and bonding. It also allows for readily accessible breastfeeding.

LLL La Leche League's (LLL's) mission is "to help mothers worldwide to breastfeed through mother-to-mother support, encouragement, information, and education, and to promote a better understanding of breastfeeding as an important element in the healthy development of the baby and mother."

Mastitis An infection of the breast tissue caused by a common bacteria that enters through a crack in the skin, usually on the nipple. The infection causes pain, lumps, and sometimes fever, itching, swelling, and discharge in the effected breast. Apply moist heat to the area for 15-20 minutes at a time and get as much rest as possible. Since it can come on very quickly, call your doctor for an antibiotic remedy if necessary. It is best to nurse through mastitis. Although your breast milk may appear lumpy or stringy, it poses no harm to baby.

MOPS Mothers of Preschoolers is a "network of women who share the common bond of preschool age children." They offer tips and discussion about parenting, marriage, health, and more.

Nursing Stool A special stool that breastfeeding moms prop their feet on during a feeding that helps to minimize lower back, shoulder, and neck, and wrist pain through helping mom maintain a supportive, comfortable position.

Oxytocin Sometimes referred to as the "love hormone," it is released by the pituitary gland when a woman's breasts are stimulated—causing the letdown reflex. It is also responsible for causing uterine contractions that help shrink the uterus back to pre-pregnancy size. Oxytocin is affected by stress and may not release when you are anxious, embarrassed, or distracted.

Plugged Duct (also called clogged duct) A sore, tender lump or knotted area of the breast caused by inadequate drainage of the breast. It usually occurs in women with abundant milk supplies because of shortened/missed feedings/pumping, improper latch, or when baby begins sleeping through the night. If treated quickly, it should not develop into mastitis. Apply moist heat before nursing, get plenty of rest, drink plenty of clear fluids, and encourage baby to nurse frequently on that side (varying positions to put pressure on different ducts).

Prolactin The hormone released by the pituitary gland responsible for making and regulating milk production. Levels of this hormone are highest at night (during sleep) and shortly upon waking. They are also high during times of physical or emotional stress.

Thrush An overgrowth of yeast occurring in a baby's mouth and/or your nipples during breastfeeding. Symptoms in baby include white cottage-cheesy patches on the inside of the lip and cheeks that aren't easily washed off; discomfort while sucking; and/or blotchy diaper rash with distinct borders. Symptoms in mom include itchy, pink red, shiny, or burning nipples; deep, shooting pain during or after feedings; and/or vaginal yeast infection. Seek medical attention if you suspect thrush, and make sure to treat both you and baby—regardless if both of you are exhibiting the above-mentioned symptoms or not. Also eat non-sweetened yogurt to help restore a good bacteria-yeast balance.

Tongue Tie a medical congenital condition that occurs when the frenulum (the tissue connecting the bottom of the tongue to the floor of the mouth) is too short and tight—causing the movement of the tongue to be restricted. Depending upon the severity of the case, this can pose a challenge to breastfeeding.

There is a simple, relatively painless procedure where a doctor can clip the frenulum to loosen it and allow the tongue full range of motion; however, doctors may prefer to wait and see if the tongue tie will affect speech before performing it. Go to http://www.tonguetie.net/index.php?option=com_content&task =view&id=3&Itemid=3 for more information.

Vasospasm When a blood vessel in the nipple suddenly constricts—causing extreme pain. Read more about this and other similar painful conditions at KellyMom.com http://kellymom.com/bf/concerns/mother/nipple-blanching/.

WHO The World Health Organization (WHO) is "the directing and coordinating authority for health within the United Nations system. It is responsible for providing leadership on global health matters, shaping the health research agenda, setting norms and standards, articulating evidence-based policy options, providing technical support to countries and monitoring and assessing health trends."

Index